SWIMMING AIMLESSLY

SWIMMING AIMLESSLY

One Man's Journey through
Infertility and What We Can All
Learn from It

JON WALDMAN

TILLER PRESS

New York • London • Toronto • Sydney • New Delhi

TILLER PRESS

An Imprint of Simon & Schuster, Inc.
1230 Avenue of the Americas
New York, NY 10020

First Tiller Press hardcover edition March 2021

TILLER PRESS and colophon are trademarks of Simon & Schuster, Inc.

For information about special discounts for bulk purchases, please contact Simon & Schuster
Special Sales at 1-866-506-1949 or business@simonandschuster.com.

The Simon & Schuster Speakers Bureau can bring authors to your live event.
For more information or to book an event, contact the Simon & Schuster Speakers Bureau
at 1-866-248-3049 or visit our website at www.simonspeakers.com.

Interior design by Dana Sloan

Manufactured in the United States of America

1 3 5 7 9 10 8 6 4 2

Library of Congress Cataloging-in-Publication Data
Names: Waldman, Jon, author.
Title: Swimming aimlessly / by Jon Waldman.
Description: New York : Tiller Press, 2021. | Includes bibliographical references.
Identifiers: LCCN 2020043443 (print) | LCCN 2020043444 (ebook) |
ISBN 9781982143947 (hardcover) | ISBN 9781982143961 (ebook)
Subjects: LCSH: Families—Psychological aspects. | Interpersonal relations. |
Infertility, Male—Psychological aspects. | Miscarriage—Psychological aspects.
Classification: LCC HQ519 .W35 2021 (print) | LCC HQ519 (ebook) | DDC 155.9/24—dc23
LC record available at https://lccn.loc.gov/2020043443
LC ebook record available at https://lccn.loc.gov/2020043444

ISBN 978-1-9821-4394-7
ISBN 978-1-9821-4396-1 (ebook)

Contents

Contents

SWIMMING AIMLESSLY

Prologue

It was a normal Tuesday in Winnipeg at the start of 2014—unspeakably cold, the streets covered in snow and sand. Slipping and skidding in the River City at peak frozen conditions is more than just a sure thing—it's a challenge, bordering on sport. The evidence is all over the highway medians: broken bumpers, tire shreds, and puddles of antifreeze are as common here as palm trees in Orlando.

Despite this, I actually find driving therapeutic. I'm one of those people who can get in their car and escape any pressure around them. During the summer I'll shamelessly blast the theme from *Back to the Future* with my windows rolled down. In winter my need for speed dissipates, but I'll still throw on my favorite tunes and sing along, head bobbing, dreaming that I'm Marty McFly, getting ready to hit 88 and jump backward, forward, anywhere else in time (well, except 2020).

This drive, however, was a bit different. I was very unsettled as I drove toward one of the local radio stations for a guest spot. Nervous to be on air? Nope. Done it at least a half dozen times in the last couple of years. Unlike some folks, I don't fear public speaking. I'd *much* rather be the guy giving the eulogy than the one who is being eulogized, thank you very much.

The year had already been a crazy one for me. With my third book—a tome on hockey collectibles—halfway done and my primary employer changing ownership, I was scatterbrained, to say the least. I took a moment to collect myself outside the CJOB studio, where I would soon tell my most personal story to the listening city of 750,000.

I arrived at the radio station as usual—about twenty minutes before I was to go on air. As always, I was overprepared, knowing the message I was going to get across, and had a rough idea of what I was going to say. It comes with the territory when you're a spokesperson for a cause; you need to be ready for whatever curveball comes your way. Emotions can run high even when you're speaking for others who are voiceless, but speaking your own truth? That's a whole other story. What was unusual was the topic—something more personal than anything I had ever experienced or spoken about publicly. It was the first time I actually had a pre-planning session with a radio host, and even with that I wasn't 100 percent ready.

As I enter the station, the receptionist tells me to hang my coat and relax—she will let me know when it's time to head into the studio.

Relaxing is easier said than done, hard at the best of times when you're going on radio or doing any sort of live performance. There are stories of NHL goaltenders who routinely vomit before game time due to nerves. I'm not *that* anxious, but still more so than usual. I study the framed articles on the wall about the Winnipeg Blue Bombers and their final game at Winnipeg Stadium, one of my favorite places as a kid that is no longer standing. Normally I'd just go through my notes or check my phone for an update or two, but this time I scramble to find anything that might distract me, ease me. No dice.

Some time passes and the previous show guest comes out. I had only slightly been listening to the broadcast on the way to the studio. For the life of me I don't know whether he was talking about the lack of snow clearance in the city, hydro problems, or other governmental issues. My mind instead is working like a dedicated engine—my eyes have blinders. Anyone from Jennifer Aniston to Barack Obama could have walked through the room for all I know—I'm getting into my zone.

Soon the receptionist motions that I can head into the booth. Gulp. The host, Dahlia, welcomes me. We do a quick recap of our previous discussion.

"So we're calling you Greg?" she asks.

It's the first time I've used a pseudonym on the radio. In the past I was always promoting a book, or a charity event. Today is different.

Today, I'm talking about a failure—the failure, thus far, to have a child. When I first volunteered to be a spokesperson for the Winnipeg chapter of the Infertility Awareness Association of Canada (now called Fertility Matters Canada), I anticipated the call from radio, but I figured it would be two or three months down the road. Instead, it was weeks. Being a male willing to tell such a personal story made me unusual. Virtually all the faces and voices of the cause were female.

And I wasn't ready to use my real voice yet.

Dahlia began the show by reeling off facts that even I didn't know at the time, including that one in six couples in Canada have trouble conceiving. I thought of Christopher Titus and his bit from *Norman Rockwell Is Bleeding*, about how dysfunctional families outnumber the "normals." How soon will more couples need assistance getting pregnant than not?

Sperm, specifically, is in trouble. For reasons scientists don't fully understand, sperm counts are down—not just in the United States but everywhere.[1] A 2019 article in *Vox* reports that in the United States, Europe, Australia, and New Zealand, counts fell by 53 percent—from 99 million sperm per milliliter to 47 million—from the 1970s to 2011. I had heard this when my wife and I got our first assessment back from our fertility doctor, but it seemed secondary to the issues we faced at the time.

Dahlia introduces me. Mic's on, ready to start telling my story to the listening ears of Winnipeg, and now to you, the reader.

Deep breath. Here we go.

CHAPTER 1

What I Thought I Knew

The first reference I ever heard to infertility was a term most kids today don't even know: test tube baby.

It was sometime in the late 1980s, and I can't remember exactly where I heard the term first—probably on the playground, or listening in while my parents watched the news. I was only ten, so I couldn't conceive (pardon the pun) of what it meant, but the slightly terrifying vision of a fetus literally sitting inside a vial immediately penetrated my psyche. I can still conjure it today.

Of course, for years it didn't occur to me to learn what it actually meant. I had more important things to worry about in high school—primarily, whether I was ever going to find a girlfriend. Social awkwardness aside, I had no real inkling of what dating, love, or relationships were, aside from watching cousins bring different partners around to family dinners until one day they were married.

But I did know that there were couples who had babies, and others who didn't. One of the latter was my mother's cousin and her husband, who lived in Montreal. Though I was plenty curious as a child, I simply didn't ask about it. It never occurred to me that she *couldn't*.

In fact, it wasn't until my wife and I started having trouble conceiving that I got a true education in how difficult having a child actually is. When we were married in 2007, I joked with my friends that I finally had a "five-year plan"—buy a house, move to full-time work, write a couple of books, go skydiving, perform a stand-up comedy act and, once I got some of that fun stuff out of the way, have a kid or two. A couple of the items on that list happened (though I still haven't had any fun with a parachute), but not the kids. On our wedding day, neither of us could have imagine the complicated road that awaited us.

And as it turns out, our experience wasn't unique.

Meet Karen Jeffries, a teacher in the New York area. While she recalls learning the basics of sex and reproduction in school, she didn't get her true education until she attempted to start having kids.

"Even when I started trying to get pregnant at twenty-nine years old, I didn't really know how you got pregnant," Jeffries says. "I mean, I knew the penis in the vagina and eggs and sperm, but I didn't know that there were only a couple of days of the month that you could get pregnant; I didn't know about the ovulation. I'm sure I was taught it, but I didn't think about it. So for our first five or six months of trying, we were having unprotected sex and I wasn't getting my period every month, so every month I thought I was pregnant. I kept taking pregnancy tests and they came back negative. I was like, 'I don't understand what's happening.'"

Jeffries attributes this to incomplete sex ed. In school she was taught that unprotected sex plus no period equals pregnancy. Now, she is hopeful that the conversation around sex and (in)fertility can expand.

"It should be talked about more in general health conversation," she says. "I wish I knew I was infertile. It would've changed things. When I met my husband and we knew we were going to be married, I would've said something like, 'I know you're the one, you know I'm the one, but I have this issue. If we want to speed it up, we might want to figure out what's going on.' We would've planned things better, but it wasn't something that was talked about."

Jeffries's experience now is affecting how she interacts with the next generation, specifically in her own family. While the New York State curriculum covers puberty in grade five and sex ed runs in junior high, she has started talking to her daughters even earlier. "I talk about it with my two girls. When they talk about having kids, I'll tell them, 'if you want, and if you can,'" she explains. "I know that sounds so negative, but I don't want them to have this thing ingrained in their head where you have to grow up, get married, and have kids; I tell them if you *want* to have kids, and I plant the seeds of *if* you can. I don't want to be doomsday, but I struggled, and as your mother I will help you. For me, that was part of the heartbreak when I was infertile. My whole life had been devoted to children, whether it was babysitting or going into education and teaching kids for the past ten years. Everything had been on a mission for children. Being realistic with kids, telling them that yes, you might get pregnant, but you also might not, is okay. It doesn't make you less of a man or woman. I think that part is okay too."

My own path was quite similar to Jeffries's. Growing up in a Jewish community and attending religious schools, there were some consistent themes in the messaging. After all, word one in the Torah (Bible) was to be fruitful and multiply.

While my overall interest in girls and women never wavered, it was a different moment that made me realize I wanted children of my own someday. When I was in high school, a new cousin was born, the first of the next generation. Watching her grow up, and being active in her life, awakened an instinct in me. I can still remember sitting with her in my parents' basement as she was learning to read and challenging her with my *Beckett* magazines, pushing her to go beyond the first reader books. I like to think I had a bit of influence on her life.

As more babies came along, I became the very involved cousin. The same happened with friends of ours who had kids first; my wife and I became unofficial aunt and uncle very quickly. Yes, there were a couple of miscarriages along the way, but those were speed bumps more than roadblocks—all of those folks ended up having kids successfully, sometimes very soon afterward.

Our story, however, wasn't going to be the same, as we learned after our first miscarriage.

CHAPTER 2

Miscarriage of Justice

One of the toughest moments of the infertility journey—if not *the* toughest—is the miscarriage.

Miscarriages are, by percentage, pretty common. Though there are different statistics floating around the Internet, some sources, such as New Life Fertility, suggest that as many as one in three to one in four pregnancies end in miscarriage (the vast majority in the first trimester).[1] So look around your Facebook profile, and you'll see that a pretty large number of your friends will have gone through this torturous experience.

Here's an important note, though: just because you have a miscarriage, it doesn't mean you are infertile. In Canada, one in six couples suffers from infertility. Some couples can miscarry one month and become pregnant again soon after. At times, an embryo just isn't strong enough to survive, or has genetic complications unrelated to the woman's ability to carry to term.

Some families, however, suffer multiple miscarriages—not only while trying to conceive naturally but also following a procedure like IUI (intrauterine insemination) or IVF (in vitro fertilization). You see, the infertility issue doesn't always mean that you can't *get* pregnant; sometimes it's that you can't *stay* pregnant. (Yet they are still often told by doctors, "The good news is, you can get pregnant.")

There is no single way to react to a miscarriage. There are certainly commonalities, but everyone will process it the best way they know how.

The stages of grief (anger, bargaining, etc.) are natural, and some will be stronger than others. But no matter what, miscarriages suck.

While research on how men react to miscarriage is sparse, some report a feeling of numbness, guilt, or anger—essentially, a brief downturn in mental health. Men, of course, don't feel the physical side of a miscarriage; for them, it is 100 percent mental, and as with many aspects of infertility, they are less likely to talk about their feelings than women.

I remember the moment my wife miscarried the first time at eight weeks, clear as day. The ultrasound doctor, who happened to be a family friend, gave a very somber "oh, no" while looking at the image on the screen beside him. I looked, saw no movement, then looked back at my wife, who was already weeping.

I didn't cry. Not because I don't, generally, but I was just frozen. I don't remember much about the immediate aftermath, other than being in the car. The strangeness was compounded by the fact that I had started a new job less than a week earlier. I wanted to be home with my wife, but how do you explain to your new boss and coworkers that you need a day off right away? (Or at least that's what was in my head; I'm sure, in retrospect, they would've understood.) This was 2009, a few years before I felt even remotely comfortable talking with anyone about infertility struggles, even though one of my coworkers, as I would later find out, was struggling as well.

The truly unique thing about miscarriage is, as I described above, how not-unique it is. RESOLVE points to several factors that can cause miscarriage:[2]

- Genetic problems. Simply put, abnormalities in the developing fetus. These can be hereditary; if your parents had a miscarriage or two (or more), there's a higher probability that you and your partner will have them as well.

- Uterus and cervix issues. These can come in the form of underdeveloped uterine linings, structural problems within the uterus such as fibroid growths, or a septum. Or the cervix may have weak muscles and cannot remain properly closed, which is crucial to carrying a baby to term safely.
- Infection. Rubella, chlamydia, herpes, and other diseases can result in miscarriage.
- Environment. Toxins in the air or ingested (through smoking, drug use, or even consuming high levels of caffeine) can result in miscarriage.
- Immunologic causes. This issue is a little more complicated. RESOLVE defines it as follows:

> One category of immunologic problems that can cause miscarriages are the antiphospholipid antibodies. Blood tests are used to detect the presence of these antibodies. If present, medication that helps thin the blood may be used. The choices are: baby aspirin (81 mg) daily, often starting at ovulation and extending into the pregnancy, and/or Heparin, a drug given by injection and used to thin the blood. Another category of immunologic causes of miscarriage are those that prevent the woman's normal protective response to the embryo.

So, pretty much everything in the above list is female-factor, but it's *exceedingly important* not to play the blame game. As men, there is little we can do to help our partners get through the moments after miscarriage, but one thing we absolutely *cannot* do is allow ourselves to think, "This is all her fault."

Instead, all your attention should be focused on your partner's well-being, and your own.

First, to the female.

Ultimately, there are many ways that women manage a miscarriage. Aside from the physical recovery, many women will go on a journey within themselves. Some might get together with friends to mourn the loss (or to avoid talking about it). Others may try a new workout program or cleanse, or take some time away from work. As men, we may not understand it all, but we don't need to—all we need to do is stay supportive. Keep your ears open, a little wider than usual, and recognize her signals.

Now, to the other important part: men's self-care. This was my first failure of the infertility journey; I did nothing to address my own pain.

After that car ride back to work, I sat quietly in my office. I knew that soon enough we had to start telling our families, and the small number of friends that we had shared our information with, what happened. I was dreading it.

What I didn't notice at the time was how little of this conversation was about me (or, at least, how I responded to the miscarriage). Yes, of course men are in many ways secondary in those early days afterward, but it's no less important that we address how we are feeling.

In 2016, a gentleman by the name of Raymond Baxter wrote a post called "Men and Miscarriage" on his blog, *The Relationship Blogger* (which was reposted on the *Sammiches & Psych Meds* blog).[3] Baxter described what he went through following his wife's miscarriage. He was so excited to be a father that he admits to not only telling friends and family but even strangers, and the miscarriage left him numb. All that eager anticipation, swept away in a matter of moments.

But Baxter shifted his focus away from himself. Like so many men, he believed he had to be strong for his partner. Unfortunately, the circumstances in his case were chaotic, like mine. He notes that while he did cry at first, he closed off the waterworks quickly because, as he had been taught (incorrectly), men don't cry. Instead, he tried to help his wife, but like so many of us, he was limited. "That day, giving my wife a hug when I got in, the helplessness I saw in her eyes, the confusion, the emptiness. It literally ripped me the fuck up inside," he continued. "Ever been in a situation where you know the person you love uncontrollably has something terribly wrong and you can do absolutely nothing to help? But perhaps hug them, even if you know that won't help one bit?"

Hugs, however, could do only so much. Ultimately, he felt helpless and numb as he shifted into autopilot mode, doing what he could to help his wife, though he knew he couldn't understand the degree of her pain.

Afterward, Baxter reflected, he began to get in touch with his emotions, but he didn't find much outside support.

"The coming weeks would suck in their entirety too," he describes. "The love, the support and the empathy would come flowing for Natalie, and I'd watch the endless cuddles and the outstretched arms from empathic friends, and I'd get a 'oh, you ok too mate?' perhaps from one, maybe two people. 'Yeah, I'm dealing' I'd say, all the while wishing I could curl up in the fetal position and rock myself crying to sleep."

Baxter's feelings of isolation, and not having his experience acknowledged, are not unusual. One of his readers, Amelia Wakefield, spoke about her own experience with miscarriage, and how her husband wasn't afforded the same support she was. "My husband and I have experienced two miscarriages and I have always wondered what it was like from his perspective," she wrote in response to Baxter's post. "At first, I'll admit that I was a bit selfish in the grieving process. I felt that he couldn't possibly know what I was feeling, and that for him the loss wasn't nearly as great.

"However, I have come to realize that he was going through it just as much as I was," Amelia continued. "In some ways, it was harder on him. People always asked how I was handling it, but never asked him. People gave me a few months to grieve and forgave me when I was just having a rough day dealing with it all, but they never gave him such a courtesy."

So now that we've established that men, indeed, do grieve a loss and aren't getting the support they need, the next step is to see that two halves of the same couple may grieve quite differently.

Adriel Booker found this out following her miscarriage.[4] In her grief pattern, she took to music, two songs in particular, to deal with her feelings. In a post on her website, Adriel explains that she would sing and cry through the lyrics and found relief. Finding her release, she shared the songs one day with her husband. When she asked her husband how he felt about the songs, his response wasn't immediate, but he offered the following: "I don't want Jesus to look after her. I wanted us to look after her."

Adriel soon came to the realization that her method wasn't going to work for him. "We would have many more conversations about our grief in the days to come, but in that moment, he needed my presence more than he needed my words," she describes. "He needed to know that I would sit in the silence and not try to explain the pain away. He needed to know that the shape of his grief was different than mine, and that was okay. He needed freedom to grieve his own way."

That small interaction helped Adriel nearly immediately. She writes that while she recognized that they as a couple grieved together, there was also that separate method her husband needed, as all men do. "We had cried together and held each other, but it was still so fresh that I found it hard to think beyond myself and my own grief," she wrote. "I was less curious about my husband's grief in the way it affected him personally than I was in understanding how it related to *us*. This small exchange helped. My perspective was widening. I was learning to better see his grief, too."

Ultimately, when you miscarry, you start to question what your next step is. Do you start trying again right away? Do you wait for the physical and emotional trauma to repair?

If you want my (hard-earned) two cents, the first thing to do is talk. Plan your next step together. You may not need to see a fertility specialist right away, but it never hurts to consult with family doctors, and a gynecologist should be your first step. At the worst, they'll tell you when you can start trying to conceive again, and if there are circumstances or hurdles to overcome first.

It also may be a good idea to consult with a family therapist or other counselor. We cannot underestimate the trauma we go through when we have a loss like this, and even though, on the surface, we may feel like we're ready to resume trying as soon as a doctor gives the okay, there is a deeper side that needs to be addressed. For instance, one or both partners may feel like there's no point in trying because it's only going to result in another miscarriage. It's worth exploring whether that feeling is based on any facts on the ground or just the pain of recent loss. And if one or both of you feel the need to just "be" for a while, and you have time on your side, consider it.

Now if you've already been trying a long time (say, a year or more), you may qualify to begin fertility tests. This is where we found ourselves, and in some ways, this is where our fertility journey truly began.

CHAPTER 3

Defining Infertility

One of the most useful ways to think about infertility is an age-old adage: know thy enemy.

Though some variance exists, most jurisdictions, medically speaking, define infertility as the attempt to conceive a child for a year without success. This is a very "simple" concept—if you can't be pregnant after twelve months of trying, you're infertile.

Oh, the air quotes I'm using? There's a reason for that: nothing about infertility is simple.

Let's start with the very basic understanding that yes, after a year of trying advice-laden guides to making a baby, you are able to see a specialist to deal with your situation. At this starting point, your medical history will be unraveled. You'll have to endure a series of questions related to your health and habits and start what could be a very long, very expensive journey to have your child.

The very first step will be to determine whether your situation is male factor, female factor, or a mix of both. Chances are that you will get a diagnosis in short order after a few tests and begin a plan to get your fertility in motion.

Or, you know, not.

You see, despite all the medical advances in the last decade, there is still a pervasive theme for many couples struggling to conceive: unexplained infertility. This is equally mystifying as it is frustrating for a couple to hear—how the heck, despite exhaustive review of medical records and invasive tests with the type of equipment that scientists years ago could hardly have dreamed of, can infertility still be unexplained?

And even more mind-boggling, how the heck is it so common? Witness this statistic, courtesy of the *Journal of Reproduction and Infertility*. In the first quarter of 2015, the journal published an article titled "Unexplained Infertility, the Controversial Matter in Management of Infertile Couples.[1] The text states, "30% of infertile couples worldwide are diagnosed with unexplained or idiopathic infertility and the problem is defined as the lack of an obvious cause for a couple's infertility and the females' inability to get pregnant after at least 12 cycles of unprotected intercourse or after six cycles in women above 35 years of age for whom all the standard evaluations are normal."

So let's go back to university for a moment. Remember that introductory assembly, where you are told to look to your left and look to your right, and that only one of the three of you will be graduating? Do the same thing now with the couples sitting (virtually) beside you; one of you will have unexplained infertility.

Lewis Black, if you're reading this, please share your finger-wagging diatribe with me, because I can't wrap my head around this.

Anyway, consider yourself fairly lucky if you get an actual diagnosis of male, female, or mixed-factor infertility. For guys, the sperm test will determine the root of your problem. For women, it's a little more complicated by such factors as ovulation, luteal phase, and fallopian tubes. Common disorders such as endometriosis will be considered before an assessment is completed and a protocol begins.

The sperm test and analysis can very easily reveal the issue, and unfortunately there are a myriad of potential conditions in men, including, as outlined by the Urology Care Foundation:[2]

- Sperm disorders. These are the most common and relate to low count, motility, or morphology. Specific conditions here can include little sperm production (aka oligospermia) or no sperm being created whatsoever, better known as azoospermia.

- Varicoceles. These are swollen veins in the scrotum. Though they affect 16 percent of males, the number increases to 40 percent of males with infertility issues. These harm sperm by blocking blood drainage and can even cause it to drain back into the scrotum, making testicles too warm for proper sperm production.

- Retrograde ejaculation. It's exactly what it sounds like: semen goes back into the body amid climax. So even if you have optimal sperm conditions, the journey to the vagina gets a big U-turn. This can be caused by any number of issues, including surgery, certain medications, or issues in the nervous system.

- Immunologic infertility. This can be any number of auto-immune disorders you may have, which result in the body literally attacking sperm, hampering movement and proper function. The UCF notes that this is fairly uncommon.

- Obstruction. Like anything else in the body, a blockage can be preventing sperm leaving the testicles. If you've had a vasectomy and are now starting to look at having a child, this will have to be reversed. Other causes of obstruction include infections, swelling, or birth defects.

- Hormones. Low levels produced by the pituitary gland could be the root issue here and cause poor sperm growth.

- Chromosome issues. Deficiencies, as well as changes in quantity and structure, can affect fertility.

- Medications. Some drugs can inhibit sperm production, including treatments for arthritis, digestion, infection, high blood pressure, and cancer. Also among the medications that can inhibit sperm production are antidepressants, which makes managing mental health an issue, one that I faced head-on (more on this later).

While the sperm test is the first you will undergo, it may not be the last. There are, to be blunt, more invasive procedures that can be undertaken to determine the root cause of male factor infertility. These can include:

- Hormonal profile. This can map out how well your testicles are producing sperm and rule out any major health concerns. The good news is this requires a simple blood test, and I emphasize "good news" because it only gets painful and more invasive from here.

- Transrectal ultrasound. Probe time! Yup, this puts a wand in the rectum and investigates ejaculatory ducts for any blockages or malformations. The technology, of course, is more often associated with pregnancy but is used for any number of internal investigations using sound waves.

- Testicular biopsy. Sorry to tell you, but it just keeps getting more painful. Cases of oligospermia or azoospermia would potentially undergo this procedure with either a general or local anesthetic administered. (Personally, I would go for general, but hey, I'm squeamish.) They'll recover tissue samples from both testicles. Along with analyzing production, there's the opportunity here to collect sperm for future assistive procedures such as IUI or IVF.

Now, as we all know, the male factor investigation is much, *much* simpler than the female factor. Some of the concerns do cross over, such as immunological issues, hormone levels, and blockages, but there are plenty of other factors for women, and the testing in general is much more invasive and painful. So, unless you are undergoing the biopsy, be appreciative that your investigation is pretty straightforward, and be sure to shower your partner with love, affection, empathy, and anything else she needs.

To give you just a small sampling of the women's tests, the UK's National Health Service website lists urine tests, blood tests, ultrasound scans, X-rays, laparoscopic investigations, and a chlamydia test (this one applies to men, too).[3] Particularly irksome (and forgive me, I have a low tolerance for doctor shows, let alone real-life procedures) are the ultrasound and laparoscopic procedures, used to detect and eliminate endometriosis or fibroids. "During a transvaginal ultrasound scan, an ultrasound probe is placed in your vagina," NHS writes. "The scan can be used to check the health of your womb and ovaries and for any blockages in your fallopian tubes." From there, other procedures will check the fallopian tubes, using a dye that is injected to see whether movement is occurring or not.

If there is a blockage, laparoscopy is the next step, which "involves making a small cut in your lower tummy so a thin tube with a camera at the end (a laparoscope) can be inserted to examine your womb, fallopian tubes and ovaries."

The unfortunate news is that, according to the US government's Office on Women's Health, 11 percent of women between the ages of fifteen and forty-four have endometriosis, so a laparoscopic investigation is a definite possibility.[4] Guys, have your best bedside manner ready, because you'll need it.

Once your infertility is defined (again, I'll emphasize *hopefully*), it's off to the proverbial races. But first, take a deep breath. The long, winding, complicated road starts . . . now.

CHAPTER 4

Starting a Journey

Every journey begins with a single step. It's a cliché, but there's a reason for it.

Many of life's journeys take men to great things in their lives. Walking into college on day one, for example, can lead to a brilliant career.

But every journey also has bumps in the road. Whether you're learning to ride a bike or attempting a triathlon (though one has to wonder why any sane individual would do this), it starts with the simplest of motions—one foot forward.

Or, in this case, one other body part forward.

The fertility journey for us, as for most couples, started with the simple agreement that yes, now we're ready to stop practicing and actually try to conceive a child. Already, we knew that certain days of a cycle were better than others, so we prepped for them and tried as best we could to set the mood. We restrained the day before the peak, and had a lot of fun for a couple of days after, but overall we didn't do anything differently than most trying-to-conceive (TTC) couples.

But it didn't work, and after the miscarriage, our fertility journey quickly turned to the *in*fertility journey.

And we were feeling pretty stranded. You see, this was the late '00s, and while the Internet was already proving to be useful for research—the likes of WebMD were answering problems long before social media proved its value—blogs were still relatively in their infancy, and Twitter was still more for news than personal venting and promotion. Facebook groups were focused on hobbies and TV shows. Instagram, which now has a very prominent infertility community of organizations, bloggers, and patients, wasn't even born yet.

We found that friends weren't that open yet, either. Everyone was either successful, assumed to be not trying, or unattached. We weren't in any support groups, and were very close-mouthed about our situation in general, save for the closest of confidants.

We didn't have much direction overall, and ultimately the only place we could turn to was the one fertility clinic in Winnipeg. Because getting pregnant in the first place was difficult for us, we were able to get into an appointment quicker than the standard twelve-month waiting window.

The first meeting with our (first) fertility doctor was anxious to say the least. The people we encountered were much what I expected—some couples, some women coming on their own—but I was worried that we would run into someone we knew, either at the clinic or in the parking lot. Located on a dedicated floor midway up a towering building, it wasn't obvious where we were headed, yet I felt like the eyes of the world were on me.

The clearest memory I have of that first meeting was the doctor's office itself. Adorning the walls and shelves, aside from an assortment of posters that you'd expect in any physician's office, were pictures of his kids and their drawings. Yes, I said to my wife once we were back in our car, I get that you want to have reminders of your family at work, but this struck me as so insensitive. You're treating people who can't have kids, while displaying your own success.

There were three steps that we talked about right off the bat, once tests were run and any immediate issues were addressed. Because we had already been using the basal thermometer and following my wife's cycle like hawks eyeing prey, the first thing we would try was fertility drugs. The second, if needed, would be intrauterine insemination (IUI), and the possible last step, in vitro fertilization (IVF). We were both determined to take the process in stride.

We were still relatively young, but the doctor did say that it was smart of us to address our situation early. I was in my early thirties at the time, and my wife was in her late twenties—years ahead of when many infertile couples would start the process.

That didn't make it any less nerve-racking, though. Plenty of our friends were already having second children while we were still trying to have number one. It was already straining those ties, as our schedules and social lives grew so different.

Unsurprisingly, it turns out we weren't the only ones who felt uncomfortable at that first appointment. Witness a blog post by Andy Thornhill for CNY Fertility, where he talked about the awkwardness of the first visit:

"I had no reason to ever be in the room for a gynecological visit and I was not ready for what I saw," Thornhill recalled. "The doctor came into the room and he was a very good-looking young man. He was asking my wife questions and asking her to prepare to remove her clothes and prepare for a very intimate but typical check-up of her undercarriage. It suddenly hit me that she was about to be medically violated right before my eyes."

Once the initial shock was over, the process was somewhat smoother. "I was very uncomfortable but as the doctor explained what he was doing and seeing I became engrossed in the process my wife and I were beginning," Thornhill continued.

Once you get past that first consult and those first exams, everything starts to become easier. It's never a fully normalized feeling, but you learn more and more about the purpose and the hope behind it. However, there is a big part of the process that does have to happen right away— the "so what do you think?" debrief with your partner after that first visit.

———

Most likely, you won't get a clear direction from an initial consult, even if you have a well-defined fertility issue. This will lead to a very emotional, probably stressful conversation with your partner, wherein both of you have the full right—nay, the duty—to say exactly what you're feeling. Think of this as the "speak now or forever hold your peace" moment of the fertility journey, because it will set the tone for everything that comes after.

And I know it's not easy to pipe up, especially if you know your views are different. One of you, for example, may want to go straight to IVF, and not "waste" time and funds for pills or IUI. The other partner may feel that if time is not an issue, it's best to try the natural way longer, explore less expensive options in the hope of not having to shell out the big bucks for IVF, or even hold off until things are more settled in your lives overall.

To have this conversation properly with your partner, though, you need to first have it with yourself. Happily, unlike actual conversations, men are pretty good at knowing what their inner voice is telling them. The difficulty comes in expressing it with sensitivity and tact.

I found, in this instance, there's a good process to be borrowed from the business world. Entrepreneur.com writer Sherrie Campbell talked about the six-part pathway to success in a 2016 article, many aspects of which apply surprisingly well:[1]

1. Awareness. Campbell states, "Always be striving for more, always be building and expanding your career and yourself as a person, not just as a success. The more you grow yourself, the more you grow the totality of your life." In infertility, you're going to find yourself forced to grow, as you delve into a knowledge base you knew nothing about (at least, I didn't) and learn more than you ever thought possible. Embrace it, even when it's overwhelming. The more you know, the more options you have, and the better chance you have for success.

2. Action. Campbell gives the age-old advice to actually get started. Plan the path to move forward in your life, and if something doesn't currently exist, draw your own map to success. In infertility, you make the map based on what you're willing and not willing to undergo. If you can't find a path by local means, you look elsewhere for solutions.

3. Accountability. Sayeth Campbell, "You have to create ways to make yourself accountable and to push through any habits of laziness or doubtful thinking. One of the ways you can do this is to share your goals with others who can help motivate you to stay on task." This one's easy. Make yourself accountable to your partner, and your partner to you. Make a plan, whether it's to get healthier to improve your natural reproduction potential, budget better to save up for IVF, or something else.

4. Attraction. Campbell comments that you will create the behavior you want and forge ahead on your goals. In other words, the more you stick to your action plan, the closer you will come to having your child.

5. Accomplishment. Campbell advises that you keep to your committed path and understand the fees and sacrifices that you will take on to get to your desired goal. "Get committed. Be willing to pay for your personal growth, financially and otherwise." Again, this reinforces sticking to your fertility plan, but also preparing honestly for the emotional roller coaster that lies ahead.

6. Authority. Campbell closes by explaining that you need to be the boss of your emotions to succeed: "You have to be the authority over your own emotions to make success happen."

In other words, you and your partner are in charge. You can listen to others, and take advice, but ultimately this is *your* game plan. Like I said before, pipe up early and often, and learn to listen well, too.

Like there are on any journey, of course, there will be roadblocks along the way. As we'll discuss in later chapters, not every procedure works the first time, the mental anguish is real, and, as we saw in 2020, forces beyond our control like Covid-19 can disrupt even the best-laid plans. But if you know what you want, set the course right, just like we did after leaving that first office, its walls covered in children's scribbles.

CHAPTER 5

Frozen in Time

As men, we are often accused of not remembering certain details. This can be a challenge when defending yourself to your mother, your boss, your spouse, or a grand jury—the omission of even the most minute detail may mean daggers being shot at you (theoretical ... hopefully).

Yet the converse is also true: the most inane comment or fleeting instance can become so embedded in our consciousness that we remember it, clear as day, even years later. Certainly, we all have that experience when it comes to historic events. If I asked one hundred people in a room right now where they were, for example, when they heard the O. J. Simpson verdict, I guarantee that more than half would be able to recount the story in full detail. (For the record, I was in tenth grade, and we were all crammed onto a school bus listening as best we could.)

Now think of something more specific to your own life. Say, your first kiss, or when you asked your special someone to marry you (especially, unfortunately, if they said no). Those deeply personal moments are just as vividly present in our minds and remain fairly true to their actuality. These are the moments that stick with you.

For the majority of men, one moment will stick out as clear as day—the moment they hold their baby boy or girl for the first time.

Infertility, however, robs you of this moment, even as you watch others celebrate it.

And this is where you start to feel so incredibly alone in your struggle—even if, intellectually, you know you aren't. When you hear friends talk about how they got pregnant on their first try, or colleagues mention that their family is growing.

The first time one of those moments happened was at the most innocent of times for me, and it was the first time that I fully felt the impact of infertility. Though we had an initial diagnosis, it was this instance that really stung, in large part because it was wrapped in such innocence. It was a mild May day; I was walking to get a haircut at a neighborhood salon. It was located on a strip like any other you'd see in any city—next door was a Greek market, across was a coffee shop and a 7-Eleven. I happened to bump into an old classmate from junior high. At that point, she had a kid and, as one would naturally do, asked if I had any. At this point, my wife and I had already visited one local clinic, but it was still early in the journey. I dodged a bit, saying we didn't have any kids yet.

Her response? "Well, you'd better catch up."

Yep. I'll get right on that . . . thanks . . . oh, and while I'm at it I'll mess with the space-time continuum and advance my kid through a couple of years, just so the kid can sit in class next to yours in middle school and experience the same awkwardness that I went through with you! (Okay, that's another book for another time.)

So why do these moments burn into our brains so effectively? Elizabeth Kensinger explained it in 2007 to Live Science this way:[1]

"Most of the time, if not all of the time, negative events tend to be remembered in a more accurate fashion than positive events. It seems like when we're having an emotional reaction, the emotional circuitry in the brain kind of turns on and enhances the processing in that typical memory network such that it works even more efficiently and even more effectively to allow us to learn and encode those aspects that are really relevant to the emotions that we're experiencing."

So there's one male myth defeated—men do have feelings.

After I parted ways with my classmate, I tried to forget her words, but just like "Barbie Girl" whenever someone says the word Aqua, I couldn't push it out of my mind. In fact, I was totally frozen. "Catching up" is something you can never do when you're infertile. Even if you adopted a kid who was the same age as those naturally born children, you'd still be behind, because you would have missed the trials and tribulations that a growing son or daughter puts you through.

I can't remember exactly what I did next, but it's a good bet I ran across the street to grab my favorite comfort food—a Slurpee. I'm not sure if I told my wife about the incident soon after or not, but something tells me I didn't, only because it was the kind of comment that is best not shared at inopportune times. Despite everything else we went through, though, it was that single moment that burned in my mind and will forever be etched as a defining moment.

Every infertile person has a version of this moment. For some, it will be the initial diagnosis, or going through a miscarriage. For Mike Heller, it was his first encounter with clomiphene, commonly known as Clomid.

Now, I do want to say that if you've had success with clomiphene, that is truly great news. If you haven't tried the drug and it has been recommended to you, know that there are some very heavy side effects. I'll get to the hard facts in a moment, but first, I'll let Mike explain what occurred when his wife used it.

I'm going to preface it like this—my wife is a hero and an untouchable queen for going through all of this shit; but man, Clomid made her crazy. I remember specifically, there was one weekend where we got a false positive and we were on the next cycle. There were friends who were supposed to be coming over that weekend and she couldn't deal with it. We canceled our plans, and she just lost it. In the throes of Clomid, she said, "I can't handle this anymore. I want a divorce and I want to move back east." Outwardly, I was like, "Okay, let's just take a minute and let's think about this, and at the end of the weekend we'll have another conversation"; inwardly I was in full sweat, full panic, like lose my mind, rip my hair out. Eventually, I was right, though. By the end of the weekend, she was like, "Sorry!" just because the Clomid ran its course and the hormones stopped flaring up. It was over—the heat at least. We're still together thankfully, went through with everything, got pregnant; but Clomid, forever in my mind, is public enemy number one.

This inflection point can come at any time. Certainly, there are obvious trigger events like baby showers and toddler birthday parties; but often, as was the case with me, it will be a seemingly innocuous interaction, something the other person likely never thought twice about.

Either way, you're changed, and it's hard to come back. In an incredible list on HealthyHappyLife.com, Kathy Patalsky compiled fifty-nine feelings that arise when you're infertile. Among those that stuck out to me was a sense of identity crisis. "I am a mom. Without a baby," she wrote.

And I really felt like I was a dad without a kid. I had several kid cousins by this time and was making sure that my wife and I were part of their lives, even going so far as to take them out to movies and giving their parents a break, or being named godparents or honorary uncle and auntie. I was the same age as the classmate I ran into, yet I felt so far behind. As much as we try to not compare ourselves to our peers, as humans, we can't help it. We want what they have. It's like when you realize you're the only single person at your tenth reunion. Even if you'd never given marriage a moment's thought, when you go into a room and everyone else is with their significant other, you suddenly feel the shift.

And here's the scariest part: that feeling never really goes away, even if you eventually do have children. You're always waiting for the other shoe to drop.

CHAPTER 6

What Causes Male Infertility

If you were in rural Ontario, near the city of London, on a particularly cold and blustery afternoon, you might have seen two surprising things.

First, you would see a male sitting alone in his car, weeping. Elsewhere, you would see another male paddling down a somehow not-frozen river in a kayak.

The kayaker I can't tell you a thing about—though I *really* wish I could—but the other man was Vince Londini.

"I don't even know what I was weeping for," Londini said on Facebook in March 2020. "I had this loss of this thing that I thought I was going to be able to do, but now I was weeping because of the uncertainty, and now we were going to have to make choices we didn't want to have to make, and explore things we didn't want to have to explore, along with a fair bit of 'why me?'"

At the time of this incident, Vince and his wife were still in their early married years. Some fifteen to twenty years later, they would still be married and have three daughters.

On that frozen day, Vince was coming home from seeing a urologist.

Though he acknowledges now that he shouldn't have gone to the appointment alone, he never imagined it would be as disastrous as it was. He had planned to head back to work, not sit hunched over in his car on the side of the road.

The urology exam was the last step in a multi-test process for Londini. When he and his wife had trouble conceiving naturally, they knew they would both need to get checked out. Londini told his wife that he would go first.

"It was a very powerful experience," Londini told me. "I prided myself on not being the guy who ignorantly insisted it wasn't his problem, and I volunteered to get tested first. It was trivial. I went into a washroom, did my thing, here's the sample, there's the test. It was a lot less invasive [than I knew her testing would be], so I volunteered."

That first test showed no sperm, but Londini's doctor wasn't confident in the results. "The first time, the doctor called back with the results and said, 'Hey, I really want you to try that test again. I don't like that lab. They came back with nothing, but I'm sure it's the lab.'"

The next step? Try another lab, which in rural Ontario meant another town. Unfortunately, they came away with the same result. "I went to a neighboring town, had the test done again, and they said, 'We're not finding anything, but that's not the end.'"

With two tests showing he had zero sperm, Vince was desperate to prove they were flukes. Unfortunately, what led to him sitting alone in his car in the middle of nowhere Ontario on this chilly day, watching the odd kayaker while breaking down, was the overwhelming feeling of grief and guilt that, indeed, he had no sperm production. It took a testicular biopsy (which alone sounds like the most painful test a male could ever go through) to confirm the diagnosis.

"That's when it really hit me," Londini said of the follow-up appointment. "In the first two samples, there was still this notion that we can fix this, there's a next step . . . I'm healthy, I'm a little overweight but I'm a pretty average guy; what on earth could be wrong with me?"

The diagnosis was unexplained azoospermia, or in layman's terms, that his semen contained no sperm. If you look up the term on Wikipedia, as you're probably doing right now, you'll find statistics that say the condition affects 1 percent of all men and factors into 20 percent of all male infertility diagnoses.

Azoospermia is one of a countless number of conditions that can cause male factor infertility. In fact, so much can go wrong en route to the egg that the more you read about it, the more convinced you become that actually achieving fertilization is nothing short of a miracle.

Let's take a step back and look at how men have been overlooked in the exploration of infertility, even though the science behind male factor has been around a lot longer than you might think.

In September 2014, MedicalXpress.com recounted one of the earliest known cases of male factor infertility, a German couple in 1881. They consulted with a Dr. Levy about their struggle to conceive. In what can best be described as an unusual practice today (though it makes complete sense in a historical context), Dr. Levy made a dozen visits to the couple and collected mucus samples from the female following sex. He then analyzed the results under a microscope and found that, indeed, the male partner was sterile.

Now, if you think that anything men go through today is invasive or inhumane, take a deep breath before reading what happened next.

Okay? Ready?

Are you sure?

Here we go.

In attempting to cure his sterility, the male went through "a tough regime of physical exercise and the faradisation (treatment with electrical currents) of his testicles." Alas, his condition was one that even such extreme measures "prove[d] unable to change."

I don't care what you're trying to accomplish—the idea of hooking up any sort of electrical device down there is just horrid. I wonder if the good Dr. Levy shouted "Clear!" before applying the electrodes to the patient . . .

Anyway, this particular procedure was just one of several pie-in-the-sky methods for treating infertility back in ye olden days, when hoops and sticks were the toy of choice. And the "science" behind infertility treatment took a long time to improve, as Dr. Christina Benninghaus explained in the same Medical Xpress article. "Knowledge about some vital aspects of human reproduction was hazy. The concept of hormones had not been developed, and the connection between menstruation and ovulation had yet to be fully understood. However, infertility was already an important sphere of medical intervention," she said. "Inflammation of male and female reproductive organs was treated with ointments, douches and massages. Women, and sometimes men, were sent to watering places to improve their health, couples were offered sexual advice, and attempts at artificial insemination were not unheard of."

There were also surgeries, Dr. Benninghaus said, and in a surprisingly progressive concept for the time, women weren't always the focus. Though some procedures, such as widening the cervix, were thought to help, at some point someone came up with the ingenious idea of testing both partners. "To spare women from unnecessary surgery, gynecologists increasingly considered the possibility of male sterility and advocated sperm testing," she said.

Still, it wasn't a widely applauded method. For one thing, as Dr. Benninghaus explained, masturbation, even for a purely empirical purpose, wasn't condoned by religious or even medical communities. And there was concern that the resulting diagnosis might be harmful to the male ego. "Men found it hard to accept a diagnosis that both destroyed their hopes of fathering children and appeared to threaten their bodily experience of potency," she said.

In the end, it wasn't until the 1960s that true assistive reproductive technology, or ART, became a reality, and the 1980s that in vitro fertilization was standardized. And even today, male factor infertility is not nearly as well known or studied as it should be.

"It goes back a long way, culturally, in how fertility has been interpreted," said Dr. Kevin McEleny, a fertility specialist based in the United Kingdom, during an interview. "It's always been assumed to be a female issue, so men have always been brought up with ideas of their own."

There are three key factors doctors look for when analyzing a man's semen, in the hilariously—and appropriately—named "swim-up test." (Sadly, what's at issue is not your ability to cross a pool to get a margarita at a Mexican resort.) They use a microscope with an ultra-zoom lens to see what's floating around in there.

Those three factors are as follows:

Sperm Count

In May 2019, ScienceDaily shared a study that suggested there had been more than a 50 percent drop in the average sperm count globally. Fifty years ago, the average was 99 million sperm per milliliter; it's now 47 million.[1] Anything below 40 million, the website reported, was troublesome; below 15 million was deemed subfertile.

So what is causing the drop in sperm count? As reported by UK-based menfertility.org, a team of Harvard researchers discovered—and I know this is going to be shocking, so take a deep breath—that the proverbial Western diet, which includes the likes of pizza, chips, red meat (processed or otherwise), grains, energy drinks, snacks, and sweets, has a major impact on sperm quantity.[2]

To prove this, the research team studied collected information from nearly three thousand young Danish men between 2008 and 2017. They compared those eating a primarily Western diet to three other groups on different diets, including:

- Prudent—fish, chicken, fruit, vegetables, and water in high quantities
- Vegetarian—vegetables, soy milk, and eggs
- Smørrebrød—cold-processed meat, whole grains, mayonnaise, cold fish, and dairy

The researchers reported the following, according to menfertility.org:

Men who followed the "Prudent" diet had the healthiest sperm overall, and they had the highest sperm count. The next healthiest diets were "Vegetarian" and "Smørrebrød." Unfortunately, men on the "Western" diet had the worst quality of sperm in the study.

Men who regularly followed the "Western" diet had a median sperm count which was 25.6 million sperm cells lower than that of men who ate healthier foods and rarely followed the "Western" diet.

Further, they found that the Western diet depleted Sertoli cells, which create a friendly environment within the testicles for sperm production.

Okay, so it's time to cancel that shipment of Red Bull and ease off the nachos. Makes sense. At the same time, though, swapping meats for beets isn't the cure that we're looking for. A 2015 study found that there are also environmental factors, including pesticides, that can impact sperm health. "Consumption of fruits and vegetables with high levels of pesticide residues was associated with a lower total sperm count and a lower percentage of morphologically normal sperm among men presenting to a fertility clinic," the study's authors summarized.[3]

Morphology

This is the actual shape and size of the sperm. Ideally, there is a round head and a long tail, big enough to propel the little guys forward. Further, as Healthline states, "the head shape is important because it affects the sperm's ability to dissolve the outer surface of an egg and fertilize it."[4]

Low morphology—i.e., a small number of well-rounded and long-tailed sperm—isn't the end of the world, as revealed by Australia's Fertility Solutions.[5] "It is quite common for fertile men to have a low percentage of ideally shaped sperm; however, when the proportion of ideally shaped sperm has significantly reduced, the chance of being fertile is lower," the company says in the aptly titled article, "So Your Sperm Morphology Is Low—Should You Be Worried?" "Even though there is a definite trend between normal-appearing sperm and fertility potential, it does not mean that a male with a semen analysis result of 0% normal-shaped sperm cannot father a child, as we only assess 400 sperm in what often are millions!"

Additionally, low morphology has no association with potential issues for the baby's health. "When assessed using the strict World Health Organisation (WHO) criteria, the morphology result is simply a marker of sperm function, which influences the sperm's chance of fertilizing an egg," Fertility Solutions continued. "It is important to remember that if an egg is fertilized with an abnormal 'looking' sperm it doesn't increase the chance of potential birth defects in any resulting children."

Motility

In short, motility is the sperm's ability to move. The standard for good motility is 25 micrometers per second, according to Healthline. Because sperm only live so long once they are outside the penis, it's important for them to reach their destination quickly.[6]

Motility can be impacted by a variety of factors. As listed by baby hopes.com, this can include overheated testicles, high stress, bad eating habits, and substance abuse (smoking, alcohol, etc.), but there can also be other underlying issues. "If a genetic defect is the cause of low motility, there is no way to correct the issue through the use of supplements, medicines, or hormones," writer Vickie Barnes states. "In other cases, low motility is caused by physical defects such as varicocele [enlarged veins in the scrotum]. While the physical problem can be corrected, sperm motility might not improve as a result."[7]

Of course, these three factors aren't the only things that can affect a man's fertility. Low libido, erectile dysfunction, and low testosterone levels can also hinder the process. Some problems may exist from birth; others are exacerbated by conditions like obesity and stress. And there are plenty of "solutions" on offer, ranging from junk mail wonder-drugs to lifestyle improvements.

One thing worth checking out is your testicular health, including varicocele. Labeled by the Mayo Clinic as "the most common reversible cause of male infertility," these swells in the veins that drain the boys can negatively impact sperm count.[8] Testicles can also be undescended, overheated (either by external factors or the body's actual function), or damaged by infection or surgery. The latter two can also affect sperm and semen production.

In my case, I received a good grade on my sperm count and morphology, but motility was an issue. As such, even if everything else was firing on all cylinders for my wife, we were still at risk of my little swimmers not being able to reach their destination. Remember—sperm can only live outside the male for a very short period of time.

Correcting my motility issues wasn't going to be easy. As I mentioned above, one of the factors that can lead to slow motility is smoking; I had smoked fewer than twenty cigs in my lifetime. I also wasn't a heavy drinker, outside of my birthday and bachelor party. So going cold turkey on Turkey Red wasn't an issue.

There were things I could do, though, and not surprisingly, the first was improve my diet.

I've never been a terrible eater, at least not since I was a teenager. Sure, I preferred burgers and fries over salads, and I was definitely a slave to the Slurpee, but more often than not, I knew my limits. Still, I was a good thirty pounds over where I should've been, and my repertoire was definitely missing a few key parts. So I set out to stabilize my eating patterns.

By this point in our infertility, my wife had started acupuncture. Though it wasn't as mainstream then as it is today, it was already gaining immense traction within the fertility sphere. I can't recall if it had been recommended to her by our fertility group, our specialist, or her family doctor, but off she went to get needle-pricked.

During one of the sessions, my wife asked the acupuncturist to see me as well. While I was admittedly squeamish about the needles, for the first time in my life, I started looking at natural means to improve my health.

First up, goji berries. If you haven't heard of them, you're not alone. Gojis, also known as wolfberries, are native to China, and in North America are most often found in dried form. WebMD cites them as potentially beneficial to people with high blood pressure, diabetes, and age-related sight issues. Gojis have long been eaten in Asia because they are believed to extend life. Naturally, gojis are high in various nutrients and antioxidants, and can help promote weight loss and healthy sleep.

All great, but what about fertility? Natural Fertility Info supplies the following answer: "In a Chinese study of 42 men diagnosed with infertility due to low sperm count and motility, the men were given ½ ounce of Goji berry a day," writes herbalist Dalene Barton.[9] "After 2 months of treatment, 33 of the men tested again had increased their sperm counts to normal or above normal averages (20 million sperm per mL of semen), and all of those men went on to father children."

Gojis were a welcome addition to my diet. Not dissimilar to dried cranberries, I would put gojis into a trail mix blend, top salads with them, or eat them on their own. Their flavor wasn't 100 percent neutral, but it wasn't overwhelming, either.

Unfortunately, I didn't feel the same way about maca root.

First, let me say that if you take maca root and can stomach it, more power to you, my friend.

Maca root originates in Peru, and is sometimes called Peruvian ginseng. It grows in harsh conditions at thirteen thousand feet above sea level, and allegedly has a three-thousand-year history as a fertility aid.

So imagine, for a moment, a desperate male seeking offspring. He has heard the legend of the maca root and its ability to increase fertility and sexual desire (which sometimes wanes when you're on the fertility clock) and travels to South America. Once he arrives, he is told of the perilous journey he will need to take to get even a smidgen of the magical plant.

Our adventurer goes to a Sherpa village, only to find that no one will guide him, given the danger involved in the climb. So he buys a donkey, rope, and other effects to get there himself.

Days later, having lost his donkey and most of his will to continue, he finally reaches the summit. His clothes are tattered and his fingers are frostbitten, but he has his canteen, and the satchel to bring home the root. Carefully, he uproots enough for his quest, and starts his descent.

Back at the village, the chief shaman preps the root, grinding it into a fine powder. In the meantime, others tend to the scars across the adventurer's body. Finally, the shaman presents the adventurer with a ladle. He takes it to his lips, opens his mouth, and immediately realizes the horrid mistake he made.

You see, maca root is quite possibly the most god-awful-tasting substance known to man. If you like cocoa, steer clear, because this will turn you off it forever. There is a hint of that sweet taste, but it's overpowered by an odd, lumpy texture with overwhelming congealment. Literally any liquid you have near it is absorbed quicker than a sponge. So unless you don't produce any saliva in your mouth, be prepared for odd lumps of what was once powder to be forming.

I wish I had known this before I went to a local natural food and supplement store. After sheepishly looking for the root, I asked one of the attendants for help. Two options came up: powder or pill form, the latter of which was about ten bucks more. You can guess which one I picked up. I asked how you consume it, and she said to take a spoonful every day.

Later that evening, I grabbed a soup spoon and tried it . . . and gagged instantly. It felt like I had accidentally swallowed uncooked raw pasta or very raw muffin batter. It took at least two glasses of water to get the taste out. Later, I tried a couple of recipes with the powder—sprinkled it on cereal, lasagna, into other flavored foods—but nothing worked. So if someone recommends you try maca root to get your boys more functional, I support spending the extra cash to get the capsules.

My other major effort was to improve my weight, and I am going to take a blind guess and say that I'm not the only male who has struggled with the scale. There've been times when I've dropped as much as fifteen pounds in three months, and others when I've gained the same amount. I've never been obese, but the pudge has been around since grade four or so, when, as my parents like to remind me, I discovered food. Until that time, I was skinnier than a hockey stick and there was a fear that my bar mitzvah would be catered with baby food. Ever since then, I've battled back and forth between a strict diet and enjoying the foods I love (particularly a Winnipeg favorite—"fat boys" from greasy burger joints).

Changing my diet was hard. I still liked those worse-for-me foods, but I cut back. I worked hard at shrinking portions, choosing healthier snacks, not eating as late at night, and going with less dense and fatty foods. With a renewed reason to push my body to its limits, I dedicated time in my weekly schedule to getting in better shape, including hitting the gym, trying out yoga, and walking our dog (when he would go outside). Shockingly, I started to feel better, and ultimately the results spoke for themselves, as a second analysis showed that my motility had indeed improved.

But remember, these were steps I took to *improve* my sperm. If I had had no sperm count at all, it would have been for naught. Why? Well, it turns out we're not sure; there hasn't been that much research done on men who do not produce swimmers.

I spoke with Liberty Walther Barnes, a sociologist and author of the book *Conceiving Masculinity: Male Infertility, Medicine, and Identity*, and her findings are shocking, to say the least.

"One of the things that I learned was that obstetrics and gynecology took root in the United States around the twentieth century, but it took a long time for male reproductive medicine to take root, and arguably it's [still] not as organized today as female medicine is," she told me. "In the United States, there is board certification for ob-gyns and then you can go on and do a subspecialty in reproductive endocrinology, and that focuses on IVF, IUI, and women's reproductive systems; and in the meantime, there's been very little attention paid to what we do about testicles and sperm."

Further, she explains, the primary research focus has been how we get the swimmers over to their destination, not how to improve the little guys themselves. And much of what has been done has not been completely validated by the larger scientific community.

"The solution has always been very female-focused," Barnes continued. "We'll take sperm either from ejaculate or testicular sperm extraction and use that for IVF—even if a woman is fully fertile—and we don't really have any medications or treatments to help men improve their sperm count. There are some that theorize that Clomid is effective in some cases and kinds of male infertility, and there's not entirely reliable data that over-the-counter supplements like antioxidants might help with sperm count, but mostly we focus on women's bodies and I would say, as a sociologist, that we just have more science—women's reproductive science is about fifty years ahead of male reproductive science."

This leaves men in a very awkward place, because we want to help—and ultimately, if the issue is us, we want to fix it, right? Apparently not—or at least that's what the doctors think.

"When I interviewed doctors, doctors said, 'Well, men don't want to see a doctor anyway, because men don't like going to the doctor, and don't like doctors poking at their private parts, so this is really a good thing that we're focusing on women's bodies,'" Barnes said.

Yep, I can say without any hesitation that I would 100 percent feel uncomfortable going to a doctor for this issue (or many others), but ultimately, if it meant the difference between having a kid and not having one? You'd better believe I would let myself be poked, prodded, or pretty much anything else. And in fact, when Barnes talked to the men themselves, this is what she heard. "When I interviewed the men, they said, 'This isn't really fair! I'm putting my wife through all of this; I'd like to take one for the team.'"

So, if fertility specialists are focused on women, where do the men turn who want to help? The answer, of course, is to a male specialist, but those are unfortunately few and far between. Barnes found in her research that those who presented themselves as experts in the field weren't always the right sources for solutions. "The men I interviewed eventually found themselves consulting 'male infertility specialists' who were primarily urologists, and even in the field of urology this is complicated because there are some urologists who don't know how to treat male infertility, and have treated men wrong," she said. "They've given men testosterone, hoping it would increase their sperm count, which, if you study this at all, testosterone actually kills your sperm production."[10]

If they aren't prescribing testosterone, Vince Londini says, they're pretty much taking the Flaming Homer approach, i.e. a concoction. Now a member of several forums on male factor infertility and a volunteer in his region for support groups, Londini sees men and couples looking deeper into the issues that surround male factor infertility than he was able to fifteen years ago, but there is still a painful lack of concrete ideas and solutions—at least, none being shared with the patient community.

"Every fertility doctor you go to has their own home-brewed, nearly superstitious mix of vitamins they want you to take. Everyone has a solution for something they swear that after they took it for three months, their wives got pregnant; but it still very much feels like it's in the realm of charlatanry," Londini says. "[Patients on message boards] post a lot more detail than I could even quote about my own lab results. They've got hormone counts and this and that. There seems to be more of an awareness of the data. To contrast, though, there doesn't seem to be a guide on how does it happen, and how do you fix it."

The issue, in Londini's eyes, comes down to the simple mechanics. With female patients, you're analyzing the reproductive parts themselves, which in many cases are much larger and easier to examine than a semen sample or individual sperm. "For a lot of male factor infertility, it's a microbiology issue," Londini says. "It feels like the male factor has a very narrow scope of investigation that is highly dependent on advanced microbiology, which you don't see happening in a hurry. Over the last fifteen years, we've seen a lot more awareness and a lot more numbers, but I'm not sure anybody *really* understands."

Case in point: D-aspartic acid supplements, also known as DAAs. As Healthline points out in an article by Atli Arnarson, DAAs have been found to be lower in infertile men than in their fertile brethren. One study found that infertile men who took 2.7 grams of supplements for three months increased testosterone by 30 to 60 percent, while as much as doubling sperm count and motility; however, as Arnarson denotes in the same article, evidence did not point to universal success. "The evidence is not consistent," Arnarson wrote in May 2020.[11] "Studies in athletes or strength-trained men with normal to high testosterone levels found that D-AA didn't increase its levels further, and even reduced them at high doses."

Arnarson also pointed to vitamin C supplements having success in some studies, but that research was currently stalled, in need of control studies.

Ultimately, even as the science progresses, we have to remember that there is no one, true silver bullet for infertility, be it for male factor, female factor, or combined. The road to fertile wellness can be aided by basic lifestyle changes, such as weight loss, alcohol reduction, and quitting smoking, but that will only get you so far. So if you are truly bound and determined to have a child, no matter what the cost, I recommend you explore widely and early.

CHAPTER 7

Debating Male Infertility Claims

Longtime fans of Fox's animated prime-time programming will surely remember *King of the Hill*.

Hank Hill and his cast of eclectic neighbors were always a good time, particularly when his son, Bobby, took a women's self-defense course at the Y. Recall the younger Hill shouting, "Let go of my purse!" and try not to burst out in laughter. Go ahead. I'll wait.

Humor aside, *King of the Hill* had some particularly insightful moments, and for men struggling with infertility there is one story line that sticks out: when Hank and Peggy tried to have a second child. This may actually be the first time that male infertility was talked about on broadcast television, as Hank's narrow urethra prevented conception, except in the miracle case of Bobby.

The episode is called "Next of Shin." Here, Hank visits a doctor after Peggy had numerous negative pregnancy tests and learns of his low sperm count. The doctor encourages Hank to do a number of things to cool down his "peaches." As one would expect, the uptight propane dealer gets plenty of ribbing from his friends when they discover his situation.

I was a teenager at the time of the episode's original airing and had never even thought about conceiving a child. Yet I suddenly wondered whether things like wearing tighty-whities, taking shots to the peaches as a hockey goalie, or sitting with laptops or other electronic devices on . . . my lap would, in fact, affect my future fertility. (Mercifully, way back then, we didn't have cell phones to worry about.)

During my first sperm test, I was found to have a low motility rate. Though it wasn't completely unfruitful, the rate was below ideal.

Ultimately, I never learned whether any of these instances had affected my fertility. But we do know a lot more now about which worries are legitimate, and which aren't.

Let's start with everyone's favorite—smartphones. Yes, they can do some wonderful things, from connecting us to the world in whole new ways to letting us scratch that *Tetris* itch whenever we need it, but they could also be causing immense damage to our reproductive systems if they are carried in our front pockets, essentially nuzzling up to our general and soldiers (particularly if we're doing the unbelievable and going commando, but more on that in a moment). Unfortunately, there is no conclusive answer as to what the effects are (or are not) on our swimmers.

For the "no, it doesn't matter" side, I point to University of Utah Health, which in 2014 published a response to a cited study that outlined the dangers of electromagnetic radiation emitted by our smartphones. One of their experts, James M. Hotaling, denied the association between cell phones and lowered sperm motility.[1] "I've never seen conclusive data that would lead me to advise a patient against carrying a cellphone in his pocket," Hotaling said, while noting that there were flaws in the study published in *Environment International*, namely that the subjects studied were already fertility patients. Further, he commented that "sperm count varies all the time, meaning from hour to hour, day to day, month to month."

The original study, from the University of Exeter, was also analyzed by Chanel Dubofsky of modernfertility.com. In a 2018 blog post, Dubofsky referenced this study as well as one published by the *Central European Journal of Urology*, which studied the effects of cell phones on the sperm of thirty-two men in 2014.[2] "The semen samples were . . . divided into two groups and one was kept in close proximity to a cell phone that was on standby mode. A call was also placed every 10 minutes," Dubofsky reported. "After five hours, the semen was reevaluated, and researchers concluded that long-term exposure to mobile phone radiation negatively impacts . . . sperm motility. The other takeaway: If men are interested in becoming fathers, they should avoid keeping their cell phones in their front pants pockets."

Now back to the Exeter study. The findings here did lean toward damage to motility. Lead researcher Dr. Fiona Mathews indicated that further research was needed; however, she did note that if you are already facing a struggle, it's probably best to back-pocket the Android.

"This study strongly suggests that being exposed to radio-frequency electromagnetic radiation from carrying mobiles in trouser pockets negatively affects sperm quality," she said in a release.[3] "This could be particularly important for men already on the borderline of infertility, and further research is required to determine the full clinical implications for the general population."

Conclusion? Let's leave it at this: if you're concerned about your fertility, don't put the gadget in front.

Another perennial debate is whether wearing tighty-whities can harm sperm production. Of course, we know the boys do need to breathe, but are boxers versus briefs going to make much of a difference? It seems the jury is divided here as well.

In 2018, NPR's Paul Chisholm talked with Dr. Jorge Chavarro, an author of a study on underwear and guys, who affirmed that yes, warmth plus balls equals damage. "Any exposure [to heat] that significantly increases temperature is likely to affect spermatogenesis [or sperm production]," said Dr. Chavarro, who (at the time) was an associate professor of nutrition and epidemiology at the Harvard T.H. Chan School of Public Health.[4] "That's the main reason we have scrotums and testes that are external to the abdomen."

Chisholm pointed out that testicles allowed to hang freely below the body are four to six degrees cooler. Dr. Chavarro's study found that the cooler environment was better, and affirmed that boxers would be the better choice. "Men who wear looser underwear had significantly higher sperm concentration and total sperm count compared to men who wear tighter underwear," he cited.

Still, Dr. Chavarro stated that his own study was inconclusive for the general population; but just like Dr. Mathews, if you have problematic situations, he advised that it's not worth the risk to go with huggers. "For most men, it probably doesn't make a lot of difference," Dr. Chavarro said. "The men who are most likely to benefit are the men who are on the border—who have relatively low sperm count."

Now these, of course, are just two of the many, *many* rumors out there, but essentially they all have the same takeaway: if you are anywhere close to being borderline infertile, it's probably best to err on the side of caution. Don't distance bike, don't spend an hour in the sauna, and for the love of God, wear a cup, even in rec league floor hockey. We men may be wired for risk and adventure, but when it comes to something this important, why take chances?

CHAPTER 8

When Advice Doesn't Help

There are certain experiences you can't advise on unless you've been there yourself. I, for example, cannot give any first-hand advice to a friend who wants to go downhill skiing, considering I've only gone once in my life (and assuredly will not do it again). I grew up in an entrepreneurial family, but have never started my own business; so don't come to me seeking input on your own venture.

I mention this because unless you have personally gone through the pains of infertility, you can't truly appreciate the struggle. Yet in speaking with associates and colleagues, the words of wisdom flow freely from the unafflicted.

Over the course of my time as an advocate, I've spoken with numerous patients, and they report all manner of not-so-helpful advice. If Rhett and Link from *Good Mythical Morning* are reading, I am hereby making myself available for you if and when you decide to do a segment I like to call "Will It Fertilize?"; but be warned, the answer in each and every one of these cases is that it has zero effect one way or another. Let's look at some of the most popular categories of useless advice!

Positions

This is one that virtually every infertile person has heard at one point or another. Somewhere, someone got the idea that women on top results in sperm leak, because gravity or something like that. I guess I could buy that argument, at least more than the next part.

You see, beyond having the woman on bottom for a better chance of sticky semen staying still, another person decided that after the deed is done (again, assuming missionary—and really, what disturbed individual came up with *that* name?), there's more likelihood of it staying if the female elevates off the bed a bit in the afterglow, again, because gravity.

If you think I'm making this up, ask Healthline. In the article "Baby-making 101: Ways to Get Pregnant Faster," scribe Stephanie Watson said the following: "No certain positions during sex have been proven to increase likelihood of conception. Yet certain positions may be better than others for ensuring those little swimmers find their way up to the egg. The missionary (man on top) and doggie-style positions (man behind) allow for deeper penetration—bringing sperm in closer proximity to the cervix."

So by that logic, you're even more likely to conceive if you buy those pills that "enhance" a male, because size matters.

Oh, wait—no, it doesn't. In fact, Watson counters her own argument just a paragraph later. After stating that woman on top has gravity working against you (again, *hah!*), she opines, "Yet standing up right after sex shouldn't reduce your odds of a pregnancy. Sperm are pretty good swimmers. Once deposited in the vagina, they can reach the cervix within 15 minutes."

And that's just the beginning.

Liquid Courage

We've talked a bit already about how alcohol inhibits sperm production, but it bears repeating here, since getting drunk is not only misguided but potentially dangerous.

I've heard from several patients who have been told to act like stupid teenagers, get drunk, and head into the back of their car (or their parents' vehicle, assuming they're still driving). No, wearing a letterman's jacket or a cheerleader uniform, with a mickey hidden somewhere, won't help you get pregnant. Let's cut that one out once and for all, with the help of Chris Iliades, MD, and his bluntly titled Everyday Health article, "Why Boozing Can Be Bad for Your Sex Life."[1]

> *Alcohol is a depressant, and using it heavily can dampen mood, decrease sexual desire, and make it difficult for a man to achieve erections or reach an orgasm while under the influence. In fact, overdoing it on booze is a common cause of erectile dysfunction.*

Clear enough? Never going to talk about this one again? Good. Let's move on.

Let's now focus on another popular liquid-based myth. Yes, that's right: cough medicine, the secret ingredient in a Flaming Moe/Flaming Homer, is said to have magical powers that will make you as reproductive as a rabbit.

Fairhaven Health responds to this supposed report, stating "the logic is easily found in the fact that it is an expectorant and is being used to loosen and thin mucus—just in a different place than the lungs," and that "any expectorant that contains guaifenesin as the only active ingredient is fine to use."[2]

Fairhaven cites a 1982 article in the publication *Fertility and Sterility* that states that taking two 200mg spoonfuls of syrup containing said active ingredient thrice a day will increase cervical mucus. Apparently you can increase this intake to four teaspoons a day if, and I'm copy-pasting this, because I don't want to spell it wrong: the spinnbarkeit—or, in layperson's terms, the stretchiness of the mucus—isn't too high. Now, this isn't as bad as our dear friend the maca root, but really, who wants to drink cough syrup four times a day?

Here's the good news: it doesn't work. Access Fertility, based in the United Kingdom, puts this myth to bed quickly. "There's (obviously) no scientific proof for this, so we can breathe a sigh of relief that we don't need to go guzzling disgusting, expensive cough syrup," writer Nicola states.[3]

Now let's look at this one in reverse: if you have a cold on heat day, can taking Tylenol Cold inhibit your chances of production? This is also a myth that needs to be busted. Cue the crash dummy, because we're about to take a visit to The Bump (and no, my brothers and sisters in infertility, you don't need to go to the website. Please, for your sanity, do not visit a site that's all about pregnancy and babies. I've done the work for you).

Writer Sona Charaipotra describes the common situation (particularly common in Winnipeg). The female partner has a cold, and has been sipping DayQuil cocktails for a few days. The basal thermometer says it's time, and come hell or high water, it's time to get to baby making. But wait, sayeth the web myth, could a decongestant do damage? Here's the slippery slope. "In theory, the problem here, if you're trying to get pregnant, is that these drugs don't have a localized effect," Charaipotra writes. "Instead, they impact your whole body, which means they're also drying out important membranes, uh, elsewhere."

Quick! Get your hands on some Robitussin to counterbalance! Or . . . maybe just see what a doctor has to say (crazy, I know). Charaipotra consulted with Janet Choi, MD, who at the time was an assistant professor of Clinical Obstetrics and Gynecology at Columbia University Medical Center. Here's what she had to say: "I haven't found any study that says this will really interfere with conception. I don't think they'll severely affect your cervical mucus—so if a patient is really suffering, I say go ahead and take what will make you feel better."

Orgasms

This is one that I heard a couple of times in discussion groups—that if a woman orgasms amid intercourse, she is more likely to conceive. Of course, no man would ever say that he doesn't want his partner to orgasm, but is any science behind this claim? No.

According to the *New York Times*,[4] women orgasm somewhere between one in three and one in four times that intercourse occurs (yes, I could say that more bluntly or vulgarly, but when one is quoting the *New York Times* . . .); so when you consider that conception is already a long shot in most cases, having a female orgasm coincide with it is about as likely as the Cleveland Browns winning the Super Bowl (or even making the playoffs).

Now even if the stars align properly (and yes, there are some who believe that a woman's menstrual cycle, including her most fertile days, overlaps with the phases of the moon), it would still just be a happy coincidence.

"There were theories that female orgasm increased the likelihood of getting sperm up into the uterus but, since then, some research has been done to disprove this theory," Dr. Savita Ginde of Stride Community Health Center in Colorado told Lauren Vinopal in a Fatherly article. "Female orgasm is its own experience, unrelated to impacting pregnancy."[5]

"You've Got Lots of Time"

I could go on and on here, but let's talk about the biggest fertility myth when it comes to men—that the male body is built to produce little swimmers for eternity. Yes, there are some cases of much older men who have impregnated their partners, but there are also people who have been struck by lightning twice.

No one will dispute that a woman's fertility declines as her egg quotient lessens as she gets older, yet many claim men can go decades and still father a child. But we don't hear much about how sperm start to change as men age.

"Male fertility generally starts to reduce around age 40 to 45 years, when sperm quality decreases," states the Victoria (Australia) State Government's Better Health Channel.[6] "Increasing male age reduces the overall chances of pregnancy and increases time to pregnancy (the number of menstrual cycles it takes to become pregnant), and the risk of miscarriage and fetal death."

So yes, we are on the clock just as much as women are. And if this were the only urban legend surrounding male infertility, we'd be in a great spot. Unfortunately, there are plenty of others. So many, in fact, I'm giving them their own chapter. Read on!

CHAPTER 9

Everything's Little with Sperm Tests

There's a pretty famous Jerry Seinfeld sketch about how when you're a kid, everything is "up."

"Clean up!"

"Wait up!"

"Hurry up!"

You get the picture.

When you're in the midst of fertility studies, though, everything is "little" for men. No, I'm not talking about the "this will only hurt a little" when they're doing examinations; I'm talking about two spots in particular that are closely tied: the little cup and the little room.

For those who haven't had the joyful experience, allow me to explain.

You see, save for some recent technological advances, men have had two options for producing their ... ahem ... sample for the famed swim-up test.

The swim-up test is simple in design and, in theory, execution. It's doing your deed solo as you might normally when your partner isn't in the mood or is not around. The only caveat here is that you can't use most lubricants, since they tend to have spermicidal ingredients. This is most definitely one of those occasions where you don't want to kill your chances of good production, so yes, in this case, dry rub means something other than seasoning you use on a steak.

You also want to ensure you are at your cleanest, so it's good to first have a shower, tidy your surroundings, and get comfortable, because everything is dependent on you, your turn-on materials (i.e., videos, magazines, catalogues, or simply your imagination), and the first of our littles—the little cup.

There's nothing more intimidating to a man than those orange or clear specimen canisters. In any other circumstance, you'd call them little. Put one up against a beer stein, after all, and it looks downright tiny. But in this particular situation, men look at that same tube and think to themselves, "Am I supposed to fill that thing?" The answer is, of course, no. Just get enough in to have a proper analysis done (the most important, by the way, are the first few drops).

To best accomplish this, men are to abstain from orgasm for two days before sample production. It's also recommended to provide the sample when you're pretty healthy. A little cough would be okay, but if you're hacking up enough to fill that little cup, it's probably a good idea to put off your sample production by a few days and cozy up to the DayQuil bottle.

Now to our other "little": the little room at a fertility clinic.

The little room is that quiet place in a medical office where we go to produce our sample when we don't want to or can't do it at home (or, on procedure day for IUI and IVF patients). The little room is usually pretty nondescript, other than the residual specter of game-day pressure.

I've been in two of these rooms along my fertility journey. There were two things that were similar: they both had chairs (though one was a very clean leather while the other was the kind of fabric you see in remnants from 1980s offices) and they both had sinks with a two-way door for collection after the deed was done.

The difference between the two, then? The "stimulation assistance," also known as porn.

One room had magazines, the other a TV with forever-running movies. (I don't think I need to tell you these weren't *TV Guide* or *SpongeBob SquarePants*.) The array in the magazine room seemed to be at least a decade old. Of course, with this magical thing called the Internet, both devices were unnecessary. Yay, phones with huge data plans!

Having said this, the little room isn't the most, shall we say, comfortable place a man can ever be to do his solo act, at the best of times. The chair could be a BarcaLounger, a chaise, or a futon, and it still wouldn't be the best place for you to sit. No matter which side of the mask debate you sit on, if there is anywhere amid the Covid-19 pandemic that benefited from increased cleaning and social distancing, it's that little room.

The male impression of those little rooms seems pretty universal. While researching for *Making Babies*, writer/director Josh Huber and his crew visited a few. "We spent a lot of time in the movie set dressing and in production design of the actual sperm collection room. I ended up taking the crew through to show them that this is what it looks like," he recalled. "Each one of them is different. Each one looks like someone ransacked a Salvation Army store."

There was one room, in fact, that Huber really took exception to. "One had a flatscreen TV that was barely bolted to the wall with an arm, and they had a porno playing on a loop. I'm not very particular about this stuff, but I'm watching it and thinking to myself, 'This is brutal. I think I need to report a rape. This is really hard-core. You need to find something really benign, like some lesbian porn or something.'

"It was all women who worked there, and I wondered, 'Did you pick this? Because this is advanced. This is *hard-core* stuff,'" Huber admitted. "They were embarrassed by it. The only thing I could do was joke around about it. The nurses were okay with it, but the guys were ashamed by it."

Even without doing a pre-deed tour of little room options, no man ever feels 100 percent ready to go in. And of course, literally everyone from the receptionist to the attending nurse to half of the waiting room knows what you're there for. So it's understandable to be a little nervous.

But this performance anxiety can actually be detrimental to the very task at hand (pun intended).

So what's the solution? There are a few options for avoiding the little room.

First, of course, is to give the sample at home (or another location, if you're into that kind of thing). Yes, you can do it in your bed, on your couch, in your bathroom (as long as your aim is really good), or wherever you want . . .

The key is, as the song in *The Pajama Game* referenced, you are going to be racing against the clock. Remember—sperm don't last long outside the body, so you'll need to rush down to a lab afterward, generally within a half hour of production; and speaking from personal experience, that part ain't fun.

For my first swim-up test, I did my handiwork at home. Going into an unfamiliar room didn't sit well with me, so I figured, where better to do it than in the comfort of my house? Bad idea, it turns out.

This was the middle of winter. While my drop-off location was a mere ten minutes away by car, winters in Winnipeg can be treacherous. Though most of us have snow tires on our car (for the southern US'ers, these are extra-grippy wheels that prevent us from slip-slidin' away into other lanes or over bridges), the accident rate is still pretty high. So delays are common, and I was doing this on a lunch break from work, meaning not only did I have the pressure to complete my exam within an hour, but to hand in my proverbial test paper and make it back to my desk in just sixty minutes.

And if you think that new parents are cautious drivers, imagine what it felt like to be carrying a specimen bottle of sperm in the breast pocket of my jacket with the heat cranked up in my sedan.

Luckily, I made it to the delivery point with a good five or ten minutes to spare, thanks to my trusty Mazda and a medical center close by. But not every region has a lot of clinics, and if you don't have a car, you don't want your little swimmers depending on the bus driver's ability to cut through traffic like a New York City cabbie.

The good news? There's another solution, per verywellfamily.com:

> *If you have any concern about being able to produce a semen sample on the day you need to for IVF or IUI treatment, talk to your fertility clinic and ask if you can produce a sample ahead of time. They can freeze it and use it as back-up, in case you can't produce a fresh semen sample.*
>
> *Ideally, your clinic should offer you this anyway. But if they don't, do not be ashamed to ask. It's better to prepare the frozen sample, and never need it, than not prepare it and possibly lose a month's treatment due to performance anxiety.*[1]

There is also progress being made on home testing kits. Among those is Trak Fertility, which can evaluate sperm counts in a matter of minutes. Greg Sommer, whose background includes working in research for point-of-care emergency preparedness applications, cofounded Trak when he realized that little was being done in the space, despite the huge need.

"From a technology perspective, we knew we could build a very precise and accurate sperm count tool that would be simple and amenable to home use," he explains. "It became evident really quickly that fertility, overall, is a big market, but men are severely underserved and overlooked across the entire spectrum of the condition."

And so Sommer and his team set out to make men more comfortable doing their part, which also helps them become a better companion on the fertility journey. "When I spoke to people, they said, 'Absolutely I'd love to do this at home, that would have been way better than what I experienced.' The vision was an at-home testing and screening tool to get over that awkwardness barrier, and it evolved from there into a tracking and improvement tool. The exciting part for us was talking with neurologists and researchers, recognizing all the things that men should be doing and can be doing to influence their sperm parameters and fertility, but that really had not been happening."

If you ask me, Trak is doing God's work. Who knows—maybe those little rooms, like the magazines, tapes, and DVDs they house, will become a thing of the past. Alas, the little cup is likely to be with us forever.

CHAPTER 10

Sex and Drugs

When you first start dating, sex is a big question mark, especially for guys.

The stereotype, of course, is that it's also the only reason guys bother dating at all. To a certain extent this is true, but it's not our fault—we're programmed that way! From the toughest jock to the most dedicated netizen, sex is a primary need for men. It can be, at times, all we think about.

And that's a wonderful thing—until it's time to make babies.

There is nothing, absolutely nothing, that kills the mood more than scheduling sex. Sex, by nature, is meant to have some sense of spontaneity, even adventure. Even if you've planned out a romantic evening and scattered rose petals (or whatever you're into), there's still an air of excitement; pleasure is the goal. And when you start trying to conceive, you're likely still having fun, at least at first; the possibility of embarking on a whole different kind of adventure is its own novelty.

But when you're facing fertility issues, the fun can go out the window—fast. Dr. Susan Feingold, a clinical psychologist who specializes in infertility, explained to *Self* that in the face of infertility, "Sex loses its association with pleasure, and often there's a loss of a sense of intimacy, loss of fun and playfulness."[1]

So let's call it like it is: sex while infertile is rarely, if ever, done for "jollies." In fact, it only happens for a scant few days a month, those being the peak times for women's "heat."

Yes, my friends, heat is real. It's damn real. It's not just for cats and dogs, either. There are actual thermometers created just for a woman to measure when she's at her most "glowing" time of the month. If there is any hope of conceiving naturally, or even with a supplement, the timing is crucial.

Babycenter.com explains it thusly:

> Timing is everything. Sperm can live for three to five days, but the egg is around for only 12 to 24 hours. To increase the likelihood of conception, it's important to have daily intercourse in the days leading to ovulation and on the day you ovulate. A good approach is to have sex one to two days before ovulation and again on the day you ovulate. That way, there's more likely to be a healthy supply of sperm waiting in the fallopian tube when an egg is released.[2]

And thus begins the schedule of sex—for many couples, the most demoralizing, unsatisfactory sex of their lives.

You see, for men, sex—or any orgasm, for that matter—is not about scheduling. Like most things men do, from taking out the garbage to shoveling snow, we do it when we feel like it. There is no "right time" (well, except when we see the recycling truck a few houses down). Male sexuality is all about the moment, which is why you hear weird stories of men being caught with their pants down in all sorts of places they shouldn't be.

Thus, the absolute worst thing for the male sex drive is to wedge it into that small window of fertility. In the days before it, the male has two options:

1. Withhold from orgasm until the appropriate day and time as prescribed by his partner; or
2. Take matters into his own hands (literally) and suffer the consequences of an enraged partner who wants to know, "What, you couldn't wait just twelve hours, you selfish bastard?"

In essence, sex becomes a means to an end, the same way working is the means of paying bills.

Now, a man may still enjoy his "work" in bed, but the sense of duty can strain even the best relationship. After all, even if you love your job, you probably don't like being pressured to perform. In fact, infertility can be hardest on the "Type A" folks, since so little is under their control.

Now that I think of it, I'm going to revise my initial theory and say that sex for the infertile couple is more like a high school exam than a job (though there is most definitely no oral portion). There's a lot of studying that happens before, there's a lot of sweating and swearing during the event itself, and then you wait two weeks to learn whether you passed or failed, thinking, "Maybe we should cheat next time?"

And just like in high school, people are more than willing to offer unsolicited advice. I'll talk about this more later on, but to be clear, no one wants to hear, "Maybe it'd work if you were on top."

Here's where the struggle gets *very* real. No matter how exact you are in your timing, how diligent in your scheduling, there's a good chance it won't work. After six months or so of trying (potentially less, depending on your age), your doctor may recommend drugs (or a bottle of schnapps, but see the bad advice chapter for more on this). Unfortunately, the likelihood of any of these "helpers" actually working is low. Back to babycenter .com for the hard-line stats:

About 80 percent of women who take clomiphene ovulate in the first three months of treatment. Of them, 30 to 40 percent conceive by their third treatment cycle.

So for this particular drug, more commonly known as Clomid, the odds are basically 1:3. At the racetrack, that's a decent chance of your pony picking up purse. In baby making, that's long-shot territory.

But more disturbing is what clomiphene does to a woman. What are those side effects, you ask? I really wish you hadn't. "Clomiphene," the same article reports, "can cause hot flashes, mood swings, pelvic pain, breast tenderness, ovarian cysts, nausea, thick and dry cervical mucus, headaches, mild depression, and visual symptoms."

Yep, clomiphene sucks.

How about another favorite, letrozole? The Advanced Fertility Center of Chicago has answers on that one, and they're not good at all.[3] According to their published statistics, "With the following conditions, we can expect approximately 15% per month for a chance to get pregnant with Femara [that is, brand-name letrozole]:

- No other fertility issues are present.
- The female partner is under thirty-five years old.
- We achieve ovulation with the letrozole in a woman who was not ovulating."

So already, that's lower than clomiphene. And the news only gets worse: when it's being used for unexplained infertility in a woman who ovulates regularly on her own, the expectations for success are significantly lower than that.

On the other side, of course, are the handful of male fertility drugs. These include Clomid, which, as University of Utah Health points out, can be prescribed to men with low testosterone.[4] "Clomiphene is used to increase the hormones released from the pituitary gland, which in turn, stimulates the production of testosterone and sperm within the testes," the clinic states. "Boosted levels of these reproductive hormones will reduce the symptoms of hypoandrogenism (low testosterone), increase sperm count, and potentially help to improve non-obstructive azoospermia."

Some research, in fact, suggests that Clomid might cure up to 10 percent of azoospermia cases. But just as in women, there are some pretty heavy side effects, including mood swings, low energy, aggression, increased hemoglobin and, perhaps most devastating, hair loss.

There are also some male-specific drugs. Among these are anastrozole, which is also used to treat breast cancer patients. For men, anastrozole can counter erectile dysfunction and increase sperm production. Its side effects can also be very uncomfortable, though: bone pain, increased red blood cell count, elevated liver enzymes, and nausea.

The good news is that anastrozole is pretty damn effective. A March 2017 study shared by the American Society of Reproductive Medicine yielded astounding results. "Approximately 95% of men with hypoandrogenism responded with improved endocrine parameters, and a subset of oligozoospermic men (approximately 25% of all patients) displayed significantly improved sperm parameters.[5] In that subset, increase in sperm parameters was correlated with the change in the T/E2 ratio, which argues for a physiologic effect of treatment."

There is another testosterone treatment for guys that has been shown to be effective: human chorionic gonadotropin (hCG). University of Utah Health reports that "the boost in testosterone production from hCG can also raise the likelihood of successful sperm retrieval in men with non-obstructive azoospermia." That's the good news. The bad news, however, is hCG requires injections two to three times a week and has some big side effects, including weight gain, enlarged prostate, and other problems.

Still, there are no guarantees. And sex can't just go back to fun and games—there's still a big schedule and a big responsibility tied in.

So if intercourse isn't working, is there any point to it? If we can't conceive naturally, should all sex stop? Of course not.

Sex is part of the glue that holds couples together, and the absence of it can quickly kill their closeness. We have to remember, as hard as it can be amid the strife of infertility, that that intimacy is what bonded us to our partner in the first place. The urge may not always be there, and there are certainly times you want to avoid intercourse, but it's important to find those pockets where intimacy and sex can happen, regardless of drugs and treatments. Beth Jaeger-Skigen, LCSW, a social worker and RESOLVE committee member, reminds couples that just because sex has to happen at certain times doesn't mean those have to be the *only* times.

"Consider having sex outside of your 'fertile' times to take the pressure off of conception," she wrote for FertilityIQ. "Avoid only having sex on a schedule. Many couples have told me that once they start infertility treatment, they are relieved to separate sex from conception. Sex can return to being solely for pleasure and connection."

CHAPTER 11

The Comedy of Infertility

If you ever wonder which of your friends are infertile, check whose sense of humor has recently taken a turn for the blue.

If they roll their eyes at your dad jokes, chances are they are infertile (or, perhaps, your fifteen-year-old daughter). If they've lost their taste for reruns of *Friends* and *The Office*, it may be because their real lives have suddenly acquired a new edge. *Modern Family*? Feh. Too tame. *Family Guy*? Getting closer.

You see, the infertility journey, with all its indignities, destroys any sense of self-censorship. When you regularly have to talk about the most private elements of your sex life, and use the words *sperm, penis*, and *vagina* with a straight face, in a clinical setting, your boundaries go from ABC to Comedy Central pretty quick. If you had any reservations about inappropriate humor, that feeling goes away with your first BFN (i.e., Big Fucking No, or Big Fat Negative, also known as the single line on a pregnancy test).

Our support group was a great example of this. When we got together for happy hour (you know, because we can), it was the *50 Shades of Grey* of comedy—mostly jokes about how "fertile people don't get it."

One particular comment stuck with me.

During one dinner prior to a group session, five or six couples converged in a pizzeria for a few slices and drinks. Somewhere and somehow, conversation turned to the little orange cup that guys are required to "fill." One of the women commented that she was surprised how little semen was produced. She always thought it looked like more when it was all over her face.

Most doctors would tell you that keeping a sense of humor amid any struggle is key to surviving it. Dr. Lora Shahine wrote about her own experience of comedy, and how she applied it to her fertility patients, on her personal blog. "As I reflected on how much better I felt after a few hours of laughing, I reflected on just how serious my days are spent with patients struggling with infertility in my practice," she wrote.[1] "So much joy is taken away from their everyday lives. Struggling to have a baby can become all-consuming. People worry about what they're eating and not eating, how much they should or shouldn't exercise, which supplements they should or shouldn't take. Planning for future vacations and career changes are clouded by thoughts of 'What if I'm pregnant by then?' or 'What if that IVF cycle doesn't work?'

"In my own practice, I've seen humor pull people through tough times," she continued. "There are the patients who brought the stuffed uterus toy to every embryo transfer, and sent me a photo of it holding their positive pregnancy test."

One couple can attest to the success of comedy for sure—Spencer and Whitney Blake. If you don't know their names, google them (make sure to include their last name, though, or you'll be taken on a road through the history of *The Hills*), because the couple created what have become landmark icons of infertility comedy: not-pregnant announcement images. "We were chatting during a road trip about 'creative' pregnancy announcements. They seemed especially popular at that time (or perhaps because we would have loved to announce a pregnancy of our own, we were more attuned to them)," Whitney explains. "We started talking about what the flip side of that pregnancy announcement is like, and the idea for our infertility announcements was 'born.'"

Creating these announcements, which included mock movie posters and memes with captions like "We spent all the dough . . . still no bun in the oven" brought out the best in their relationship and helped them through a very tough time, much as it did for Spencer earlier in his life. "Laughing *during* a struggle (and not just looking at it in hindsight) is crucial. For example, my dad passed away when I was in college," he says. "Such a devastating loss obviously comes with countless tears, but my mom, siblings, and I used laughter in that instance when appropriate. Looking back on memories of my dad made us smile, and I felt he would be happy to see us remembering the good times. Humor has helped me deal with and move forward from infertility, disappointing news at work, or just a plain ol' bad day."

And here's where there's an interesting dynamic. With their censors down due to the nature of infertility being so invasive in your private life and exposing your bedroom (or bathroom, or kitchen table, or . . . well, you get the picture), the comedy among women seems to get more to that "dirty" level that women tend to turn not just their cheek, but their entire body, away from. As IFLscience reviewed, women were more often than not turned off by crude humor. Using two blue jokes as their testing strip, the researchers found one hundred women and provided them with said gags, as well as clean jokes, and associated them with dating profiles of random men.

The result? "The finding that women prefer ostensibly benevolent humorists and that there is a general motivation to engage in benevolent humor use across contexts is consistent with previous research," the authors stated; or, if you prefer layman's terms, clean comedy is the go-to for the majority of women.

It would definitely be interesting to see what the results would be if that study was done with one hundred infertile, medication-sick women who had gone through three IVF cycles. My guess? Well, after most respondents replied, "Who cares if he's Danny Tanner funny or Bob Saget funny—does he have working sperm?" you would get the feeling that the crass jokes are more accepting. Trauma tends to numb us to many experiences, so being able to enjoy a darker comedy certainly goes hand in hand as you seek enjoyment; and if there's anyone who's mastered the art of infertile comedy, it's Karen Jeffries.

Yes, this is the same teacher I talked with earlier about the lack of infertility study in today's curriculum. Like many superheroes, Jeffries has an alter ego—she's the brains behind *Hilariously Infertile*.

Jeffries has done it all in her infertile career—she's a stand-up comedian, a blogger, a meme expert (or is that memer?), and an author. Part of the appeal, of course, is that she gets down and dirty in a language that you wouldn't necessarily expect, yet it's the one she's spoken her whole life.

"I've always been really inappropriate. Like, *really* inappropriate," Jeffries admits. "I've always been the person who talks about the stuff that no one wants to talk about. Even if it came down to farting, I was always like, 'Why aren't we talking about this?'"

So when Jeffries and her husband discovered that they were having trouble conceiving, she went straight to that dark place that most normal folk wouldn't go.

"I was like, 'Oh my gosh, this is all about penises and vaginas, and it's hilarious!' Don't get me wrong—I cried and I had those moments—but there were so many things that I was like, 'Yeah, this is funny.'"

What Jeffries quickly recognized was that her sense of humor was very well suited to men. She shared a sensibility with more male comedians than her female peers, notwithstanding the welcome recent infusion of Ali Wongs and Amy Schumers to the comedy world. Jeffries classifies that sensibility, quite correctly, as Grade Seven humor. (Who am I to argue with a teacher?)

"Reproductive humor is pretty much that—it's for a seventh-grade boy, and I think it goes along very well with my sense of humor and my husband's sense of humor. We just think it's really, really funny."

Her husband should be applauded, not only for finding such a force of nature to marry but for being the motivating force behind *Hilariously Infertile*. As Karen's biggest cheerleader, he pushed her to pursue the blog and the book, and created a monster that he could never have seen coming. While I didn't ask if Mr. Jeffries was a sailor, it turns out he did blush.

"After I wrote the book, I shared it with my husband and he said, 'This was not the type of book I thought you were going to write.' He thought I was writing a self-help book. He looked at me and said I had ramped it way up—*way* up. I asked him if it was funny and he said, 'It's funny, but it's very, *very* detailed, raunchy, and inappropriate.' But that's how women are."

Okay. Time out. Flag on the field.

Aren't women the "fairer" sex? Aren't men the dirty creatures who laugh at poop jokes and the mere mention of the word *vagina*?

"Sometimes this is lost, mostly on men, that women aren't more raunchy than men, but what me and my girlfriends talk about is way worse than what my husband and his guy friends talk about. We'll go out for dinner and talk about discharge, sex . . . we'll talk about anything under the sun in an open restaurant. We don't care. Men? They just talk about sports and finances."

So the reaction she got from her friends and family was the reverse of what one might expect.

"I wasn't nervous about his reaction, because he knows me and we joke around all the time. I was more nervous about his guy friends and how they were going to respond to the book," she says. "They were with us when we were going through it [infertility] and they were fine, but I was more nervous about what they were going to say about the book and if they were going to give me a hard time about this. In the end, all of my husband's guy friends have been so beyond supportive."

So now we have an interesting dichotomy: women are more likely to talk about their sex lives, but men's sense of humor originates in middle school and many times doesn't evolve past it. The two coming together, thus, would seem to make the shared experience of infertility that much easier to have laughs about . . . right?

Unfortunately, Dr. Tracey Sainsbury worries that most couples won't be able to share the funny as easily as Karen and her husband. In fact, she thinks joking around about the experience could even do damage. "I think less than five percent of the couples I've worked with would agree [that comedy is the infertility language]. At times, if you try to make light of something, it can be taken so badly," Sainsbury says. "I think the key thing is no couple is the same, and every individual has their own baggage."

So how best do we, as men, approach the situation? At first, the best thing we can do is tread lightly. Don't go full-out Sam Kinison right away. Look at the situation and consider how well (or not well) your partner can handle lightheartedness about such a serious topic. If you've been paying attention throughout your relationship, you probably already know the answer.

The bottom line, though, is that laughter is one of the best medicines when approaching infertility. It's therapeutic to chuckle in stressful times. If you can't discuss the topic directly, find levity elsewhere. Maybe turn the channel away from *CSI* and more toward TBS. It can improve your mood and conversations, which never hurts—because if there is one thing infertility does, without fail, it's challenge a marriage in ways you never thought possible.

CHAPTER 12

Standing Strong in Marriage

Hey man, are you and your partner having difficulty conceiving? Do you feel like she isn't the same woman you married? Does she seem obsessed? Emotionally fragile? Always sad? Angry? Don't worry, it's all normal!

—Erica Berman, PhD[1]

This is how Dr. Berman opened her 2013 *Huff-Post* article, titled "When Infertility Affects Your Marriage." Obviously, it's a generalization, but I think most women navigating infertility would admit that they feel this way at least occasionally. Some will go further, saying that the inability to conceive totally changed them as a person.

Make no mistake—men have the same reaction. We may not display it outwardly, but infertility makes us rethink everything.

The reality is that the man or woman you married or agreed to have a child with may be a different person today. This can be a serious challenge, because so much of beating the fertility odds depends on keeping your relationship strong.

Whether you are married, common law, or in another sort of partnership, there is so much that depends on the success of your relationship as you struggle through any difficulty; but when a couple struggles to have a child, it can be a major killer, especially once you begin the procedures to hopefully have a child.

One study in Denmark found that, after an unsuccessful fertility procedure, couples were three times more likely to separate.[2] The study followed 47,500 women, whose average age was thirty-two, for roughly seven years, with the first subjects chosen in 1990. By the time the study ended in 2007, more than one-quarter of the subjects were living alone or divorced. One-third were childless.

There's no question—infertility messes with marriage. There are all kinds of stress-inducing factors, including lack of agreement on how to proceed, anxiety around timing, and the serious side effects that accompany many fertility procedures. Fertility problems can be damaging not only to the partnership but to each individual's sense of self.

Dr. Berman emphasizes that the most important thing for men to understand is how common these mood changes are. She writes:

> *The men supporting these women are often surprised and unprepared for their reaction. They often assume it is a sign that something is wrong with their partner. They worry that the woman they married will never reappear. They often don't understand why their partner is so upset about something that is totally beyond her control. They don't understand why she can't be happy for others' successes. To try to 'fix' the problem as best they can, many men will simply try to reassure their partners that it will all be OK. But in reality, he cannot know that this is true and these types of statements end up making women feel even more emotionally isolated. They assume that their husbands' less extreme reaction is because they are less invested in having a child.*

So how do you avoid the trap of being together in the battle, yet very individualized in your approaches? Well, unsurprisingly, the unifying principle is the same as for successful marriage in general: communication, communication, communication. When men go into their shells, as we tend to do, it can create an uncomfortable situation. The key, as author and journalist Kate Brian points out, is to talk instead.

"Sometimes women do report that their male partners aren't engaging with their fertility problems and treatment in the same way they are themselves, and that's why talking openly to one another is so vital," she says. "Often it's not a lack of commitment from the male partner, but is more about different ways of dealing with difficulties. Communication is vital, and it's important to create time and space where you can both be honest with one another about the way fertility problems are affecting your lives."

This is easier said than done, however. Just as communication styles vary widely, so, too, does the language used. Perhaps, then, to further Karen Jeffries's point, the best method is to use the humor that's now exposed amid infertility to better talk with your spouse. "You definitely need to have that emotional support and going through all those relationship things and not putting blame out—you're in this together—but I think the best way to go through it is with comedy. Everyone's always asking, 'Is laughter the best medicine?' and my answer is, 'Fuck yeah!'" she says. "Infertility is so sad. It's not funny, but if you can focus on those funny parts, as opposed to those sad parts, you'll get through those sad parts a lot better, because you'll be saying, 'I had the roughest time at my appointment and I saw this guy walking out of his exam room and I just started laughing hysterically.' All those things you're told relationships have to have is good, but comedy and lightheartedness is very important."

Can too much humor, however, be a bad thing? Remember what Tracey Sainsbury believes: that few couples she has encountered would agree on this path.

So what, then, is the path to better communication between partners? There isn't one universal right answer, explains Brian. "There is no
one-size-fits-all solution when it comes to improving communication,"
she says. "Some couples may be very open with one another from the
start, but infertility is such an intense experience that there are often
communication issues."

Part of the underlying problem is that most adults still have only a
rudimentary understanding of what happens when you start trying to
have kids. Sainsbury cites a study by Fertility Network United Kingdom.
While the primary focus of the study was on the suicidal thoughts that
sometimes accompany infertility, it also explored how the very nature
of our thoughts and being change the moment that we lay our cards on
the table and announce to ourselves and our partners that it's time to
start trying for a kid. Any successful parent will be different from how
they were pre-baby (unless they have a superpower that allows them to
drink until midnight and still manage the kids fresh as a daisy the next
morning at the ungodly hour of 5:30 . . . not that I speak from experience
or anything).

When infertility rears its ugly head, however, that anticipated change
gets delayed, and your thinking can go a bit sideways. Your partner may
not understand, and conflict results, even though it's no one's fault.

"The theory is that your unconscious goes through a paradigm shift
when you're ready to try to become parents," Sainsbury explains. "If you're
a woman and you're not trying to be a mom, your unconscious archetype
is of a domestic goddess, a sexual being, a career woman, etc. But the
minute you're ready to try to conceive, it's like Mother Earth and you're
put here to make babies and that's all that matters. And as a human, you
become a catastrophic failure if you don't [have a baby]. The man's unconscious, before trying to conceive, is often focused on being a provider,
and that Earth Mother is telling him that caring for your partner means
reassuring her, 'Don't worry, it's going to be fine.' So there's a mismatch in
what's going on in the unconscious. Neither's wrong, but unless we un-

derstand what's going on unconsciously, as well as consciously, we can try so hard to say the right thing and it ends up making things worse."

At this point, many couples will seek third-party guidance, which Brian sees as beneficial as long as both parties are buying in.

Of course, as Brian told me in an email, there is sometimes reluctance about seeing a counselor, particularly from men. They may see it as admitting weakness, when in reality it is often a sign of strength to acknowledge a problem and try to address it. All couples counseling offers a safe space for partners to talk about their feelings and experiences with someone who will listen and support them. And a specialized fertility counselor can help couples communicate effectively in a very challenging situation. I know many couples who described it as a lifeline.[3]

Every couple is different, and what works for one may not work for another. The key is to find support you both feel comfortable with. Either way, the absolute worst thing you can do is play the blame game. Whether your infertility is female factor, male factor, or a combination thereof, you're in it together, and if the bulk of the woe (or the work) falls on one person's shoulders, it's a recipe for disaster.

Unfortunately, I witnessed this very occurrence in mid-2020. In a men's infertility support group on Facebook, one member, who shall remain anonymous, posted the following:

> *My wife is shouting at me no end these days and I seriously can't take it anymore. As she keeps telling me she's in this position in life because of me. Which is totally true. I've put her through 3 IVF cycles and we've had 2 miscarriages. Again, due to me. It's true she has had to change her work life majorly because of me.*
>
> *We were supposed to try for another cycle in a couple of months, but the way things are, I really don't want to do it. I just want some peace and to not have to walk on eggshells.*
>
> *I'm sure time will heal and things will improve, but for any-*

one that has divorced over this—what were the telltale signs for
you that divorce was imminent?

Ten days after the thread started—an eon by social media standards—good brothers, myself included, were still trying to talk the OP (original poster) out of his funk. But no matter what we said—sharing our own experiences, suggesting that professional help may be the best avenue—the member was inconsolable. He was defeated by the very partner that he needed to depend on for comfort and support.

The OP eventually went quiet, without sharing the outcome. But another member posted with a harsh reality—that despite their best efforts, he and his wife could not make their marriage last. "I ended up divorced 3 years ago, after 8 years of trying," the respondent wrote. "You may get to a point where it has taken such a toll on the marriage there is nothing more you can do; the infertility experience is irrevocable.

"After much reflection that marriage never would have worked without a natural born kid, I wish I had those years back to have more fun, and would have avoided years of agony."

This is the unfortunate reality of infertility. Not every problem will be solved; not every issue can be addressed and cleared up. Infertility not only crushes future dreams and desires—it can quickly endanger what you already have. And this leads us to the most insidious aspect of infertility: its toll on your own mental health.

CHAPTER 13

Problem Solvers

He: Damn it, just let me help you! You keep going on and on about this and you don't seem to want to do anything about it!

She: I'm not asking for your help! It's not a problem that I want to fix . . . there's nothing here to fix. Will you please, just for once, stop offering me advice??!!! That's not what I'm asking for!

He: I don't get it! What on earth do you want? What am I supposed to do with that?

She: I just want you to listen! You seriously don't get me. You don't listen to me!!

He: AAAAHHHHHH!

This is how Simon Niblock started a blog entry titled "Men & the Problem with Being Problem Solvers."[1] It's a scenario that might sound queasily familiar: the insistence of the male on "helping" his partner, when instead of creating a solution, he is only exacerbating the problem.

The throes of infertility are particularly torturous for this problem-solver mindset, since so little is in your control. Moreover, you should be concentrating much, if not all, of your efforts on helping your spouse—in whatever way she tells you she needs. This is just one of those areas where men cannot—I repeat, *cannot*—be problem solvers.

This, unfortunately, doesn't sit well with most of us, since we're programmed for action from virtually the start of life. As Niblock reports, "Men frequently say that they feel utterly useless and unhinged if they can't fix a problem. When men are attending to some type of responsibility, fixing, performing, or solving a dilemma, they know they belong."

And this is a major issue for an infertile man's mental health. When we're desperate to be the fixer-upper and can't do things in the correct turn, we freeze. The logical part of our brain, which is shouting, "Ask for help, you stupid, determined male!" is still drowned out by our instinct to be the all-purpose handyman.

Witness the experience of another problem-solving male, Rick Wamre. In 2006, Wamre penned an article for the *Oak Cliff Advocate* about a situation involving his wife forgetting to pack, in his words, "feminine hygiene products," and his trying to be (again, as he puts it) Solution-man.[2] Amid his journey, Wamre makes an admission:

> *Since I had already spent my allotted "ask for help card," I was*
> *on my own to make the decision. I remembered my wife once*
> *saying that wings were silly, so I eliminated all winged products.*
> *However, I was still faced with an ocean of options. It was then I*
> *became a victim of advertising. I replayed every horseback-*
> *riding, tennis-playing, how-your-period-is-freeing television ad*
> *I could remember and selected a familiar brand, sans wings. I*
> *returned to the hotel, wet from the rain, and presented my wife*
> *with the spoils of my adventure. After telling her of the ordeal,*
> *she thanked me and said, "a tampon would have been fine."*

Of course, Wamre should be applauded for seeking assistance once without batting an eye; but male pride stepped in and told him not to do it again. If his wife was on FaceTime at this point, she surely would have rolled her eyes.

I don't point out Wamre's follies to shame him; rather, this is the perfect example of a male admitting that he was wrong and coming forward with his story. In his own way, Wamre has made it acceptable for men to admit that it's okay to not be problem solvers—or, at the very least, that you don't have to solve every problem solo. Given that 2006 was ancient history in technology terms, Wamre may not have had a mobile phone with which to text or call his wife, who likely would have pointed him to the right product in the drugstore, particularly as he stood in front of the gigantic selection of pads and other products when, as she told him when he returned, a tampon would have sufficed.

The reality is that no matter how much we try to rewire ourselves, we can't. Believe me—I've tried thousands of times. The best advice I ever got was to simply shut up, listen, and support, and while I think I've gotten much better at it over the years, I inevitably slip up, and ultimately pay the price for it. But don't despair; if full reprogramming isn't an option, there are still ways to modify the approach and make your actions more effective.

Michelle Roya Rad, a psychologist, discussed the characteristics of a "good problem solver" in a 2013 article for *HuffPost*.[3] In her article, Roya Rad lists ten key facets:

1. They don't need to be right all the time;
2. They go beyond their own conditioning;
3. They look for opportunity within the problem;
4. They know the difference between complex and simple thinking;
5. They have clear definition of what the problem is;
6. They use the power of words to connect with people;

7. They don't create problems for others;

8. They do prevention more than intervention;

9. They explore their options;

10. They have reasonable expectations.

Most interesting, to me at least, is item number 7, because when we try to solve problems, as Niblock found, we often (inadvertently) create a larger issue. Roya Rad describes this point as follows:

> They understand that to have their problem solved, they can't create problems for others. Good problems solvers who create fair solutions make a conscious effort not to harm others for a self-interested intention. They know such acts will have long term consequences even if the problem is temporarily solved.

I think every male reading this book can recall a time when we've turned a molehill into a mountain by losing sight of the consequence of our actions.

So how does all of this play out in infertility? Unfortunately, unless you are a fertility doctor and therapist yourself, you can't solve the problem; but there is good news for husbands who may feel left out of the decision-making process: your voice and opinion matters. In 2019, *BMC Women's Health* published results of a study conducted with 246 Chinese women undergoing IVF treatments between 2014 and 2015.[4] While 92 percent reported that they shared "decision-making tasks" with their doctors, 52 percent also said that they would also share the decision-making with their husbands, and an additional 46 percent said they trusted their husbands full-out to make the decision on behalf of the family.

Now all of this is a good starting point, but you must still understand that you can't do it all on your own. Even if your partner comes to you and says she trusts you to make the right decision, you have to constantly consult. Given the forever changing fertility landscape, it's impossible to know which path is the best without going through a few steps.

So what's the best thing that we, as pigheaded men, can do? Be present when our partners bring up the idea of going into a support group, be it in person or virtual; go to that extra doctor visit or to see a family therapist. Consider it a research initiative if you must, but being present in these situations will help you be the most educated partner you can be. Not to mention it might help ease your mind about the decision being made, if it's not entirely up to you.

After all, the reason men enjoy the problem-solving role so much is because it gives us a measure of control. We like to feel that we are in charge of our own destinies, and that when a roadblock comes in our path, we can either stop, change paths, leap over that block, or smash it to bits with a sledgehammer (I'll give you five guesses as to which most men would prefer to do). Infertility is a roadblock in some ways, but rather than being a simple barricade it's a giant chasm dug out from the street in front of you and, at least at first glance, it's the only road from one town to the next.

Ultimately, the best problem solvers know that they don't have all the answers, and as hard as it is, the best thing we can do is ask for help. Seek the advice of others and talk about our issues.

One problem, though: if the first people we talk to outside our partners would be our friends, how do we do that when men rarely talk?

CHAPTER 14

Men, Mental Health, and Infertility

In the end, infertility's greatest impact on your health will likely be mental, and as you've probably heard, most men aren't great at dealing with mental health challenges. This chapter would be less than one hundred words long if I left it at that, though, so let's dig a little deeper.

First, it's important to recognize that even without infertility, six million men in the United States alone are dealing with depression. Though the number of women who suffer is greater, this is still a huge quantity, and likely an undercount when you consider, as the Mayo Clinic points out, that men tend not to recognize or seek treatment for depression.[1]

Of course, it's not a big surprise that the disappointment that comes with infertility might impact your overall mental health, but you may be surprised at the depth of that impact.

Consider this commentary from Dr. Esmée Hanna of the Centre for Health Promotion Research at Leeds Beckett University. In an interview with iNews in the UK, she said:

A recent statistic suggests that around 42 per cent of all those with infertility issues have considered suicide. That's probably a shocking statistic to those without personal experience of infertility, but one that I personally am not at all surprised to hear, and that's why I think it's so important that support options are in place for men, as well as women.

Let that sink in for a moment. More than one in three individuals who is going through infertility actually *contemplates* ending their life.

Now, add that suicide is four times more prevalent in men than in women.

Scary? You bet.

I certainly counted myself among the depressed, and went so far as to contemplate suicide on multiple occasions. The stress and anxiety (and I don't need to tell you that anxiety rates are exceedingly high right now as well) associated with infertility is demoralizing, to say the least. So many questions, so many paths . . . it was like reading the *Choose Your Own Adventure* books again, only this had much higher stakes than being eaten by a dragon.

That's not to say that my depression was entirely due to infertility. Like many people, I was already struggling with mental health by the time we discovered we were infertile.

Growing up, I often felt the effects of depression. It was numbing. I had trouble with normal social situations, including making friends, and felt academically and physically behind my peers. (Okay, in the last case, being five foot five, I wasn't expecting to play varsity basketball, but the continual cycle of being picked last for every team certainly didn't help.) I was slower and less agile than most of my counterparts, with a healthy dose of social awkwardness, and over the years it took its toll.

By the time I graduated high school, I definitely felt like a loner, and for the most part, an outsider. Then again, in a small community school with a graduating class of nineteen, it's hard not to feel that way. You're always under a microscope, at one of the most vulnerable stages of life.

This was the mid-1990s, before the Internet had truly opened up, and even having a cell phone was unusual, so reaching out to a teen help line was not something I considered. There was also still a stigma around mental illness, so I was unable to really find that pathway out.

Throughout this turmoil, without recognizing it, I was finding outlets to channel my pain. I was deeply involved in my youth group and student council, and hobbies like sports cards and video games. So rather than dwelling on myself and overthinking everything, I remained fairly level-headed, all things considered. The suicidal thoughts just felt like part of me, and I didn't truly recognize just how much I needed help.

Once I reached university, things started to improve, but the despair would still hit me from time to time. At a certain point, I became convinced that I was dealing with seasonal affective disorder (SAD), a condition I could now find clinical research on (thanks to the advent of a brilliant service called Netscape). Rainstorms, for instance, broke me down to the point where even getting out of bed was hard. They still do today. Snow I can handle, but that bone-chilling heavy rain you get on many fall evenings in Canada is literally putting a wet blanket on me. Other times, the early winter darkness would level me.

But later in life, I would learn that what I thought was SAD was really only an indicator of a larger mental health issue, and having a predisposition to psychological struggles meant that I was poised for a full-on downward spiral once infertility arose.

And boy, was there ever a spiral. Performance, in every aspect, crumbled. My brain, at times, felt like it completely shut down. I no longer enjoyed some of my favorite things, like floor hockey, and stopped doing them altogether. Many days, I barely could get myself out of bed, let alone go about daily tasks; and anything I did was done so poorly that I'd look at it later with a clear head and wonder why I had even bothered. Even today, the effects of this low point linger. I hesitate to call it PTSD, but the symptoms are similar. A flash of feeling different, out of sync, can plunge me into the dark corners of my mind and make me almost blank out at times.

As a fully grown adult at this point, I struggled to find good coping mechanisms, mainly because it felt like everything I *could* do wasn't what I *would* do. The social outlets weren't as easily available as youth groups in high school, and going to the gym regularly got harder, as my study life changed to working life. Holding down a regular job, plus freelance obligations, meant twelve-hour workdays, which left little time for anything else. I didn't turn to alcohol or drugs, but I did isolate myself in front of video games for hours, which is its own kind of dangerous. Yes, annihilating thousands of robot drones can be a good way to vent, but more and more often I found myself plowing away at *NBA Jam* or *Street Fighter II* rather than going out with friends or talking with someone on the phone (in ye olden days before WhatsApp, you used this mechanism to . . . okay, getting off topic).

But what really suffered was my relationship with my wife. I hadn't dated much before I met her, but I had been on enough bad dates (another story for another book) that I knew she was the one I wanted to spend my life with. Unfortunately, my unresolved mental health issues meant I wasn't always the greatest boyfriend or husband. What had started in high school and crept through university without being attended to was starting to affect my partnered life. I didn't pay much mind to it, because I was too busy working, and by the time infertility hit, I was downright terrible to deal with. I consider myself fortunate, though. Somehow, my wife put up with me, for which I am eternally grateful. Her patience was a godsend.

What actually happened, as Tracey Sainsbury describes, is that the skeletons in my closet came back to haunt me. The self-esteem issues that plagued me in high school came back in a big way, as did other feelings of inadequacy. As Sainsbury describes, the compounded feeling I felt is quite normal amid infertility. "Fertility has a habit of retraumatizing every other trauma in your past that's connected to family," she explains amid an interview over Skype. "If you've been in a relationship in the past and hoped to have a family, that can be retraumatized by struggling to conceive. If there's stuff in your own family that's been difficult to manage or there's a situation where you were unable to control or influence the outcome, that can be retraumatized. Things that have happened far in the past can feel very present."

Ultimately, what I realized was that no amount of threatening or cajoling, by my wife or anyone else, was going to get me out of my mental hole. I had to do it of my own volition. I had to learn to accept who I was, not who I thought I should be; and this was exceedingly hard to do. I've always had that underlying feeling, as I think many of us do, that I wasn't good enough or didn't deserve good things in life; when I did have a success that I rightly could have celebrated, I downplayed it or looked past it to the next step. No, I never shot a hole in one (though I did break a club once . . . that's sort of the same thing, right?), but I did manage to do some cool things like write for magazines and newspapers I read growing up, and eventually write some books. Yet none of it made me feel whole.

So what did I do? I let myself be vulnerable. My wife and I went into counseling, and I explored individual therapy as well. Ultimately, this led me to going on antidepressants, which I was admittedly scared as all heck to take; not because of the stigma, necessarily, but because I felt ashamed that I needed to take a pill to feel "normal."

The vulnerability hurt. How bad? Imagine taking a punch from Tyson Fury to the exposed stomach while his boxing glove is laden with glass. Oh, and you haven't eaten for days. That's how bad it hurt. Opening up, knowing full well I was going to be a sobbing, crying mess, was terrifying, and I had to coach myself through it.

Of course, my wife was by my side, but I felt like I needed to take it a step further and explain my at-times odd behavior to my friends, opening up about my mental health and the new steps I was taking. Their reaction was, for the most part, positive, but a few couldn't accept it. Some thought the pills would be temporary (I wish they were); others deflected the conversation to somewhere less personal (I'll give you three seconds to figure out which gender did that).

The most rewarding moment was when I expressed myself in a lengthy post on the infertility support group we were now part of. I danced with Facebook's character limit for a good half hour before finding something meaningful and succinct enough. I knew my burden was not unique, and I thought it needed to be shared. What I found was that I not only connected with my new tribe (though naturally, 90 percent of the online group was female), but my expression had inspired others to talk with their spouses and themselves.

After all, this was back in 2013, before apps focusing on mental health were readily available. Some, like 7 Cups, were starting to pop up while I was going through the first round of my mental health journey, but the larger conversation was nowhere near what it is today.

In the absence of this outlet, many of us turned to social media. While message boards were passé, Facebook groups were in their boom period. Though I was hesitant to say anything using my real name, I looked to these outlets for posts that would make me feel less alone and any helpful articles that might aid me. When I finally wrote my own post, I was near tears, but I knew I was speaking straight to those who would listen most.

When I look back now, as I continue to work on being a better man, I'm so glad I finally kicked myself hard enough in the ass to snap out of it. I know that sounds ridiculously self-serving, but one of the factors perpetuating humanity's mental health crisis is how few of us actually acknowledge our problems, much less actively look to solve them.

So why is mental health so hard for us to talk about in the first place?

Part of the issue is purely cosmetic—unlike a broken bone or a permanent physical limitation, mental health issues aren't visible, and the treatment isn't simple. One can't put a brace on and undergo physiotherapy to fix a mental health issue. Even with the myriad of medications available for patients, finding a proper "cure" for depression and anxiety is hard, and often the mix includes group counseling, individual therapy, new activities (with the emphasis on *active*), and other elements.

If this sounds like a lot to tackle, it is. But not tackling it can be even more costly, in the end. Mental illness drains energy, time, and bank accounts. Today, many companies have recognized this reality, and are actively striving to improve their employees' wellness by providing healthy snacks or offering increased leave options; but a decade or so ago, that wasn't the case.

Now we get into a vicious cycle, since there is a correlation, of course, between mental health and substance abuse. One study by the *Journal of the American Medical Association* found that 37 percent of alcohol abusers and 53 percent of drug abusers had at least one underlying mental health issue.

Alcohol, cigarettes, illicit drugs. These are all things that not only perpetuate mental health issues but also can drastically harm one's fertility. We'll use alcohol as an example, and for this I turn to addiction.com. In the article "Five Substances That Can Affect Fertility," the writer (referred to as Staff), states:

> *In a 2005* Fertility and Sterility *study, researchers compared sperm quality in moderate drinkers with that of 66 alcoholic men, who drank about six ounces or more of alcohol daily, or nearly so. The researchers detected abnormalities in the alcoholics' reproductive hormones and found that their sperm count and motility (how well the sperm could move through the female reproductive tract) were significantly lower compared with the non-alcoholic control group.*[2]

So there, in plain letters, is your snappy retort to the "if you guys got a little drunk . . ." advice.

According to the same article, other substances that can affect your fertility are tobacco, marijuana, heroin, and cocaine. So, that pretty much covers the gauntlet.

Oh, and you can add to that list mental health issues themselves. In a blog post titled "Infertile Men and Mental Health Issues" on his website, Dr. James Elist discussed an investigation that revealed a tie between anxiety and a negative impact on fertility.[3] "According to a study reported in the *Indian Journal of Medical Research*, investigators suggested that chronic mental stress can negatively affect the quality of sperms and semen," Dr. Elist wrote. "Based on the analysis of semen obtained from 27 volunteers, it was observed that high mental stress is related to high serum levels of superoxide dismutase as well as the enzyme catalase in the serum; directly contributing to the poor motility index of sperms and overall concentration of spermatozoa in the semen."

Now compound this with a relatively new phenomenon—the struggle to be a male.

And no, I don't mean in comparison to women. This is a battle unique to today's male, where "traditional" definitions of masculinity are running up against a society that is pushing males to open up more—to be in touch with their emotions and express them; to allow themselves to be vulnerable.

Consider the plight of Phil Christman, for example. In an article for the *Hedgehog Review*, Christman relives a painful conversation he had with two women in his workplace (presumably face-to-face, pre-Covid-19) who openly push at stereotypes of men.[4] "'Men don't have to think about how they look,' says another coworker, also a woman, and I nod again," Christman wrote. "Then I realize, days later, that the reason the statement is still bugging me is that I am literally never not sore from the gym, because I am so concerned with looking a certain way."

Christman later identifies another issue, after a transgender friend asks him what it's like to "feel at home in your body." His internal answer?

"The only answer I can come up with is that I never feel at home in my body. I live out my masculinity most often as a perverse avoidance of comfort: the refusal of good clothes, moisturizer, painkillers; hard physical training, pursued for its own sake and not because I enjoy it; a sense that there is a set amount of physical pain or self-imposed discipline that I owe the universe."

By no means is Christman alone. John Haltiwanger, in an article for *Elite Daily*, looked at the downright insulting phrase "Be a man!" and synonymous forms.[5] "Every single male in the world has heard these three words in some form or another: 'Don't be a p*ssy'; 'grow a pair'; 'man up,'" he writes. "We hear these words when we don't live up to prescribed notions of masculinity. After all, men are supposed to be tough. This mentality is doing more damage to humanity than most of us likely realize."

Further, Haltiwagner opines that "there's a pervading sense of powerlessness among men, and it's a consequence of their inability to express themselves. Most men would likely not admit to this, and perhaps aren't even cognizant of it. Yet, these are precisely the sentiments forcing men to seek other means of feeling powerful."

Bingo. If you aren't allowed to embrace your feelings and confront your weaknesses, then you will use other forms to express your might. As you can imagine, this can turn very, *very* unhealthy.

So, if men, according to stereotypical legend, are supposed to be tough as nails and as hard as stone, and this is hammered into us at every corner, both by other males and by females, as Christman demonstrates, how do we break the cycle?

While some would take it to the basic drill-down of being in touch with your "feminine side" (which in itself is an offensive term, implying that women are gentle and tender and less powerful), there is a much more basic, and accurate, interpretation: be in touch with your inner self.

Yet this seemingly simple directive has plagued both men *and* women for years. Diving deep into your own consciousness and wading through the weeds of your psyche, facing damage head on, and admitting weaknesses is so critical to coming out the other side healthier. One patient, who went just by Rob, talked about his first experience with therapy, and how he "almost" allowed himself to open up completely, on the blog *Sick Not Weak*:

> *For me, an "almost" is defined as a welling up of emotions to the point of almost uncontrollably bawling my eyes out, but then, as I have done so often before, stifling back those emotions and tears until those emotions and tears are no longer visible to the outside world, all part of that "mask" that many wear.*

Rob described how he kept getting close to opening up fully, but it was too painful. "I really wanted to lay on the couch," he wrote, "but thought to myself, 'nope, not going to lay on the therapist's couch, that's how all the flood gates open.'"

The feeling is one we all experience, whether we're talking with a therapist, our spouse, a friend, or a support group. As much as we *want* to talk, our competing instinct—to protect ourselves and keep our vulnerability to a minimum—is equally strong. No one likes to cry, yet we all need to sometimes. No one likes to go through that feeling of being at the brink of vomiting due to our high emotionality, but those of us who have been through it come out the other side with some sense of a path to betterment, or at least to how we can better cope with our anxieties and deficiencies.

Does it feel better to talk? In the short term, no; but in the long term, yes. Taking that first step is immensely hard, but take it from someone who has gone down the path more than once—you come out on the other side feeling like, at long last, there is a sense of direction.

And when you're on an infertility journey, you sorely need that direction.

CHAPTER 15

Avoid Being a Fertility Fool

The coronavirus has had some devastating impacts on individuals and families; but in the midst of a dire situation, communities bonded, as we do in today's social media–rich era, over memes and viral jokes.

Most of these were genuinely funny, such as Michael Scott holding a coffee mug emblazoned with "Toby Spread Covid-19." Others celebrated the forced isolation as an introvert's paradise.

Not all were funny, however. One of the common refrains was how there was bound to be a baby boom nine months from the start of the lockdown.

Yep, that's how it happens. You stay indoors for a couple of days, get bored, have lots of sex, and boom—instababy.

Thankfully, the joke quickly dissipated, but it was yet another example of how thoughtless, even throwaway words can negatively affect a patient. The same takes place annually on April Fool's Day, when social media-ites who are either single, newlywed, or already swimming in a pool of many children post a pregnancy announcement, only to be followed by "April Fool's!"

These sorts of posts really do damage, more than you think. Witness a Global News story in 2019.[1] Fertility Matters Canada volunteer Vidya Ledsham talked about the situation she faced when she had two such "announcements" appear on her Facebook feed. "When you're facing infertility, pregnancy announcements are difficult. Even when they're coming from people you love, and they're true pregnancy announcements," Ledsham told the Canadian broadcaster. "When other people get to announce their pregnancy, you [wonder], 'When will I?' Then to have someone joke about it, you deal with all of these emotions only to find out it's a joke. It's such a flippant comment for some people, but it's not [always] easy to get pregnant."

Lisa Rosenthal agrees. In a blog entry posted just days prior to April Fool's Day 2019 on the Reproductive Medical Associates of Connecticut's website, Rosenthal commented about the false pregnancy posts she sees on Facebook.[2] "Not resonating? Maybe it's a little bit funny? If so, try this. Instead of 'I'm having a baby', take away 'baby' and insert 'cancer' into the joke. Can you imagine?" she wrote. "'I have cancer. Ha, no I don't! April Fools! I don't have cancer!' How would you or anyone react to that? How is having cancer in any way funny?"

Those sentiments are felt fully by women on the journey. Conversations in infertility groups online around April 1, every year, are of the same remorseful tone—a mix of "if only they knew" and "bad form."

But are men more likely to brush off such witticisms? I can't speak for all men, of course, but those posts irked me, to a point where I couldn't take much more. I can't remember exactly what the comment was, but I actually messaged a friend who made a misinformed joke on Facebook about fertility and how easy it was to get pregnant. My cohort, of course, was immediately apologetic after I messaged him privately, which was of course what you'd hope for in a response; but as Rosenthal notes, there is a distinct lack of recognition of how many people are suffering, including men.

I remember another post in a general male support group on Facebook. One member, who had been trying with his wife to conceive for eight months, posted a simple question about natural means to increase his sperm count. Among the oh-so-helpful responses were "Just relax and f**k" and "Get another dude's stuff and then inject it in yourself."

Yep, real medical professionals here.

These sorts of comments explain why men don't bother piping up in the first place. If a support group isn't a safe space, where we hope to speak without getting blasted by stereotypical guy comments, then what's the point in talking?

So, if you are one of the lucky "breeders," take heed of this lesson: don't be a fertility fool. Help your brothers who are in need—and don't make them feel worse than they already do.

CHAPTER 16

The Religious View

After I began speaking openly about my infertility struggles, a member of my community asked me to speak at a Jewish education event.

I've always had an easier time speaking in front of strangers, but Winnipeg's Jewish community is small. Chances were that if I didn't directly know an audience member, they would know my parents, my sister, my cousins, or one of the above; be a distant relative themselves; or know me through my involvement in Winnipeg Jewry. So, the idea of standing up in front of a room of thirty to forty familiar faces, most of whom knew something of my story, was nerve-racking.

I worked on the speech for a few weeks, doing a ton of research on my Judaic background as it related to infertility. When I arrived, PowerPoint ready, I was greeted by a packed room . . . of empty chairs.

Was I shocked? Somewhat. I had spoken with a few community members privately about their fertility journeys, and my family was getting a lot of support with our struggles, so I was pretty disappointed that no one showed up to talk about such a prominent problem.

It was as clear a sign as I had seen that religion and infertility don't always mix. I'd known some couples who struggled with their beliefs when it came to infertility treatments, but I was spared such conflicting feelings myself.

Religion and I, to put it bluntly, didn't have the greatest relationship. After going through various sects for schooling, I'd had enough God talk by the time I left home. By no means had I abandoned my faith, but I enjoyed bacon as much as I did gefilte fish. I didn't join the Jewish fraternity in college, nor the culture-based group on campus. I did seek to date Jewish women as much as possible, and married within the faith, but I wasn't looking for an ultra-devoted partner. Our wedding was performed in a synagogue, by my rabbi, but we attended services only on the High Holidays, bar mitzvahs, and the days of mourning.

So when it came time to seek guidance about my infertility, I didn't do what many of my peers did—consult a rabbi or other religious leader. My experience was more cultural, insofar as one of the agencies that my wife and I approached was the local Jewish Child and Family Service. If we were going down the path of adoption, we did want to explore the possibility of adopting a Jewish child. More on this later.

I could never have predicted that in my post-announcement life, religion would suddenly become more present.

In preparing my semi-sermon, I learned that Judaism isn't the only faith whose relationship with infertility is complicated. Elizabeth Hagan, a multidenominational American pastor who struggled with infertility herself, wrote in a *Time* op-ed, "while many of us might think of turning to religious leaders for comfort or encouragement, unfortunately the words we often hear back from them are less than reassuring. Many couples say that their faith communities are the least safe place when it comes to their fertility woes—a place that regularly hosts child-oriented rituals and ceremonies, and that celebrates Mother's Day and Father's Day, elevating the stories of biological parenthood above all others."

Of course, most churches and synagogues are also very committed to educating this next generation on the correct path. It's a sound business strategy, after all.

So how does religion view infertility? For that, I turned to gotquestions .org, a very catchy title (for those pre-millennials who remember the Got Milk? campaign, of course), which provided the following insight from the Judeo-Christian perspective:

> *Artificial insemination, also known as intrauterine insemination (IUI), is a medical procedure in which a man's sperm is implanted in a woman's uterus at precisely the right time and in precisely the right location in order to increase the chances of pregnancy. While it is usually used in conjunction with fertility medicine in women, this is not always the case. Artificial insemination is different from in-vitro fertilization in that fertilization occurs inside the woman and in a more natural way, while in-vitro fertilization occurs outside the womb, and then the fertilized egg(s) are implanted in the woman's uterus. Artificial insemination does not result in unused or discarded embyros. Artificial insemination does not have as high a success rate as in-vitro fertilization, but many Christians view it as a much more acceptable alternative.*

Okay, doesn't sound too ba . . . hey, wait a minute, something's not sounding right here. Almost like . . . no . . . IVF isn't a sin, is it?

> *The Bible nowhere discourages anyone from seeking to have children. The fact that artificial insemination does not have the moral dilemmas of in-vitro fertilization would seem to make it a valid alternative.*

Okay, so IUI is kosher according to this website, but IVF gets the big no?

I had to look a bit deeper into what was being cyber-preached, so I went to a few other websites.

One of the first answers in my Google search came from Ron Conte, a Roman Catholic theologian. Conte addressed the question in a straightforward blog post titled "Is IVF a Sin?" Right off the bat, Conte states, "Yes, IVF—in vitro fertilization—is intrinsically evil and always gravely immoral. It is always a serious sin."

Conte expands thusly:

> *The conception of at least several embryos is accomplished in the petri dish, and only some embryos are selected for embryo transfer (ET) to the womb. Other embryos may be frozen, for later possible use. The remainder are routinely destroyed. More than one embryo is created so that the ones showing the most vigorous growth can be implanted. This type of selection—of which human persons will live and which will die—is an abomination and a grave crime against humanity.*

So there's one resounding answer to the "when is a baby a baby" argument. But Catholicism, we know, has always taken an absolutist view. How about other faiths—were they any more forgiving?

It didn't seem so. Take Sikhs, for example. The BBC reported on one dichotomy that exists within this religious community. Sikh families place a high value on having children and alleviating the suffering of an infertile couple; yet there is also the belief that infertility is the path laid out by a higher cause. "Most Sikhs believe that all life is sacred because it is given by God," the article states.[1] "Therefore, many Sikhs interpret infertility as being the will of God. It may be considered God's way of showing [the infertile] that they are not meant to have children."

And if donor sperm is required, get ready to be accused of living in sin. "Some Sikhs believe that AID (Artificial Insemination by Donor) is a

form of adultery, because it introduces a third person into the conception process."

So how about Islam? Well, you're not going to have much success
there, because just testing is considered an unholy act, according to the
study "Psychological and Social Aspects of Infertility in Men: An Overview of the Evidence and Implications for Psychologically Informed Clinical Care and Future Research."[2] "In Muslim communities," authors Jane
R. W. Fisher and Karin Hammarberg wrote, "religious beliefs make infertility assessment and treatment particularly difficult for men because
masturbation is proscribed." The same philosophy, to be fair, is present in
Judeo-Christian circles, where there is a belief that the act is "wasting the
seed," as I was once told. So there's your euphemism du jour.

Happily, the book *Contemporary Bioethics: Islamic Perspective* offers
a bit of a different perspective. In the chapter "Assisted Reproductive
Technology: Islamic Perspective," authors Mohammed Ali Al-Bar and
Hassan Chamsi-Pasha write, "Artificial reproduction is not mentioned in
the primary sources of Shari'ah; however, when procreation fails, Islam
encourages treatment, especially because adoption is not an acceptable
solution. Thus, attempts to cure infertility are not only permissible, but
also encouraged. The duty of the physician is to help a barren couple
achieve successful fertilization, conception, and delivery of a baby."[3]

Perhaps surprisingly, some major religions are very clearly on the side
of ART. Witness, for example, Hinduism. "Children have always been
important since time immemorial and the continuity of the family unit
has been of major significance in Hindu culture," reported Fertility Plus.[4]
"Indian mythology is full of stories about what couples have done in the
past to overcome their problem of infertility. Hindu Religion has tried to
understand the natural hurdles infertile couples may face to fulfill their
social obligations, and made alternatives available."

The emphasis, it seems, comes from the strong, simple obligation to
have children. "Each individual is bound by Dharma to produce one child

who must perform the annual ceremony of Shraadha (offering oblations to ancestors)," Fertility Plus continues. "This child is a Dharma Putra. The Shraadha offerings enable the ancestors to nourish themselves in their abode—Pitr loka. Without a Dharma Putra to make that offering, ancestors suffer torture, hunger and thirst on Pitr Loka."

So, if you're ever looking for a motivation booster, there you have it.

And it isn't just Hinduism—Buddhism also takes a positive approach to ART, says buddhisma2z.com.[5]

Buddhism does not object to this procedure as such because it helps to alleviate a particular type of human suffering (the distress of not being able to have children) and it does not contravene the third Precept. However, there are several aspects of IVF that could be ethically problematic. Some religions object to IVF because the sperm is obtained through masturbation, which they consider to be a sin. Buddhism does not raise this objection, firstly because while it does not consider masturbation to be skillful, it does not see it as evil, and secondly, while it may be unskillful, in this case the intention behind it would be a good one.

If you're not lucky enough to be Hindu or Buddhist, you may not find the full-throated support you're seeking from your church elders. But I still believe that most people, whatever their creed, can understand the pain of wanting to become a parent. So if you're a person of faith, and it's important to you to share your journey with the community, reach out—chances are there are others there going through the same thing, with many of the same questions. And if not, you'll know it's time to look elsewhere.

CHAPTER 17

Remember the Grandparents

There's a famous dad joke that goes something like this:

A new father calls his mom and dad from a hospital to tell them that their new grandchild has arrived. The new grandmother and grandfather are excited, of course. Grandmother rushes to the car while Grandfather goes to his study, takes out a book, and makes his way to the car.

At the hospital, the grandfather and grandmother meet their new grandchild. While the grandmother holds the baby, the grandfather pulls his son, the new father, into the hallway.

"Son," he says with a tear in his eye, "congratulations. We're so happy for you. I wanted to give you this. It's been in our family for generations."

The grandfather gives the father a book titled *101 Dad Jokes*.

The father looks to the grandfather and says, "Dad. I don't know what to say . . . I'm honored."

Grandfather replies, "Hi, Honored, I'm your dad."

Now, dad jokes (including those that end with the line "The Aristocrats!") are a time-honored tradition, even if we only gave them a name in the last decade or so. Dads, by nature, are cornball when the time calls for it (and often when it doesn't). Generally, they do a very effective job proving that dads aren't as funny as they think they are (unless your last name is Seinfeld, Brooks, or Reiner). Happily, they also cement a bond between generations of men that few other aspects of fatherhood can.

In today's world, where men of different eras often have radically different experiences of marriage and fatherhood—not to mention religious beliefs and political leanings—it's important to seek out common ground. After all, no matter how much we fight with our parents in adolescence, most of us grow closer to them (if we're lucky enough to still have them) after we have children of our own. Yes, that constant mantra of "one day you'll understand . . ." suddenly rings very true.

After all, this isn't just a parental threat—it's also an eagerness to go through the wonderful experience of being grandparents.

Today, many would-be grandparents are worried they may never get there—stepping in to lend a helping hand, spoiling that new generation, and most importantly, seeing their own children as parents.

In 2016, Jeannette Kupfermann spoke about this fear to the *Telegraph*.[1] Though neither her son nor daughter had evidence of infertility, they both got married later in life and, at the time of the interview, had not yet borne children. The sudden recognition that she may never be a grandmother began to hurt. "I felt an enormous sadness at first," Kupfermann told reporter Anna van Praagh. "You're meant to go through certain cycles at certain points. I used to think that until I had grandchildren, I was out of sync with life. I can only describe it as an emptiness."

I certainly felt this longing from my own parents. While my sister got married later in life, I was a spry twenty-seven years old when my wife and I were wed.

What unquestionably made it harder on my parents was their relationship with their young (grand)nieces and nephews. Being the second-youngest of my first cousins, all of whom were at least five years older than me, meant that the next generation was well underway by the time of my wedding in 2007 (three of these cousins, in fact, had parts in the ceremony).

Because my parents were relatively young, and physically able to play with those kids, they became honorary grandparents to some. They visited their homes, celebrated their birthdays, and hosted them at our cottage north of Winnipeg.

For a while, this "substitute grandparenting," as it were, satiated their desire for grandkids of their own. But naturally, they still longed to see me and my sister on the path to parenthood.

My wife's parents did, too, of course, but the circumstances were different. Unlike me, my wife was among the oldest of the five cousins in her generation, and the only one in a committed relationship by the time she reached her midtwenties. And amazingly, she still had grandparents of her own. At the time of our first pregnancy, she had two grandmothers and one grandfather still alive. Not long after the miscarriage, we lost her remaining *zaida*.

The passing definitely shook our families, and we both felt the effect of having one less great-grandparent to share our first child with. Still, with two great-grandmothers, there was the urge to keep pushing forward, and with both in their eighties in families who had a history of long lives, the likelihood was that a future child would be part of a four-generation family.

Which, of course, prompted comments from one grandmother that she wanted to push a stroller before she pushed a walker.

Having said all this, it's fair to describe my situation as atypical. Eventually, after our daughter was born, my sister had kids as well. Often, it happens that one sibling will have children on the "regular schedule"; so if you and your siblings are already prone to the "mom always liked you best" rivalry, relationships can get strained pretty quickly. Most grandparents don't want to add to any hard feelings between siblings, so they're quickly put in an awkward spot. Shady Grove Fertility, which operates several clinics across the US, described the situation in one of their blog posts:

> *Very often parents of an infertile couple feel caught between their infertile child and their "fertile," sometimes pregnant, child(ren).*

Naturally, both offspring may expect to rely on their parents for
emotional support at this significant time in their lives. While
this is a realistic expectation, many parents may, for a variety of
reasons, end up providing more support to the "pregnant" child
than the infertile couple. Sometimes this happens when a parent
is more knowledgeable about providing support around preg-
nancy and parenthood issues than about infertility. Other times,
it may be that pregnancy and grandparenthood is a happier,
more enjoyable experience, while infertility brings sadness, loss,
and a variety of negative emotions.[2]

So if you think sibling rivalry was hard on your folks when you were little, imagine what it's like when your stations in life start to differ.

Additionally, a sister or brother might reasonably expect that the infertile sibling and the sibling's partner still engage with their new nephew or niece. But if they are insufficiently sensitive in their requests, Shady Grove reflects, it can also put the (grand)parents in a difficult spot. "Sometimes they feel trapped in the middle—or worse, their children demand they declare a specific loyalty or that they take sides," the clinic states on its blog. "It is important to remember that parents still set the tone for family interactions and values, even in adulthood, and must refuse to take sides."

So as we can see, splitting time between the fertile and infertile becomes a tricky balance—and that's assuming that the infertile couple has shared their struggles with their parents, at least somewhat. "The infertile offspring may not have asked for parental help, keeping infertility a secret, or may have asked for assistance that is impossible to provide. Many parents become paralyzed by their child's pain and feel helpless to know what to do," Shady Grove notes.

I can certainly relate. My parents are terrific, yet that same overwhelming feeling of failure that I struggled with throughout our journey made it hard to even talk to them about the experience.

So how can parents be supportive? There are a few easy ways: be mindful of invites to child-centric events; wait for your child to bring the subject of children up, rather than continually asking about any updates (in other words, don't smother); perhaps even consider attending a group session with your son or daughter.

What's also important is to investigate the general emotional temperature in your family. Both men and women want the family to continue growing, of course, but a man may feel more responsibility to ensure this happens, perhaps due to the tradition of the last name being carried from the male down.

One man I spoke with, Vince Londini, mentioned the genetic line and the ways he felt he was failing. "You can be okay, then you can be reminded that you're the end of your family line. It's always important to you—this notion of genetic connectivity—which we're always enculturated with," he says. "We have this default notion that genetics governs belonging; but then you have this feeling of 'I can't do that. There won't be any more of me.' To most of us, genetics might as well be magic, but we have this notion that we are what we are because of our genes, and now we can't pass that on. It was a huge emotional package for me."

Beyond this emotion, Londini and his wife identified another key area of hardship, while deciding whether to share the news of their struggle with their parents:

> We knew we would begin to invite advice, and we weren't ready
> for advice. We didn't know what we were going to do, but we
> knew we would resent if someone began staking out their opin
> ion, and pushing us to one thing or another, or telling us not to
> do anything.

And in truth, this is perhaps the most common problem when it comes to family and infertility. The instinct of any parents is to help their child when they are in need. In some cases parents have learned to step back and let their children find their own way—but others, well, you can't spell *smother* without a certain six letters.

Yep, you've got it. Perhaps you've even used the term yourself. I have, as my mom pointed out amid her toast during my wedding. Ultimately we can thank Adam F. Goldberg for bringing about the "Smother" into the mainstream—the overprotective, over-involved mother that many of us grew up with. And in the case of infertility, the Smother has lots of ideas, most of which she saw on TV or heard from one of her friends.

Mike Heller feared that the smothering would start when he confided in his own mother. "You don't want to talk about it. We didn't want to share with our families because that turns on questions: 'Did you do this, did you do that, what do you think of this, what do you think of that?'" he explains. "Especially my mom—she's an interrogator, she's a steamroller, and she takes on all of our problems and feels like she needs to fix them because it makes her feel bad, so it makes her feel better by making us feel better."

And that last sentence is the key to why our parents get so involved. Our pain inevitably hurts them, too, and they can't help but want to help. Remember, their situation is not so different from ours: they want grandchildren. Heck, many people will say they look forward to being Grandma or Grandpa more than Mom or Dad.

No one, outside of the couples themselves, are as invested in the success of a fertility journey. So let's try to be patient with the would-be grandparents, even when they're on our last nerve. After all, they're just loving us the best way they know how—which is what parenthood is all about.

CHAPTER 18

Not-so-Happy Father's Day

Father's Day. A Hallmark holiday? Sure. A true opportunity to show Dad some love? Perhaps. A painful day for the infertile man? You bet.

Though it's never quite achieved the cultural cachet of Mother's Day, and it often gets lost amid the rush to summer holidays, you can't discount the importance of Father's Day for men, especially those who don't get to experience it properly.

Father's Day is just over a century old. Its origins, as one might expect, are fairly humble, but very meaningful. "In May of 1909, Sonora Smart Dodd of Spokane, Wash., sat in church listening to a Mother's Day sermon. She decided she wanted to designate a day for her dad, William Jackson Smart," wrote Remy Melina in an article on livescience.com.[1] "Dodd's mother had died in childbirth, and Dodd's father, a Civil War veteran, had taken the responsibility of single-handedly raising the newborn and his other five children."

Surviving Father's Day, on the surface, may seem easier for the infertile male, since the plethora of Father's Day commercialism pales in comparison, by far, to that of Mother's Day. Where the May holiday has celebrations at every restaurant, sales on flowers, and just about every imaginable way to fete mother dearest, Father's Day is considerably more quiet.

Regardless of the public promotion, however, it hurts like hell when you can't celebrate it.

I didn't pay much mind to Father's Day when our infertility journey began, probably because it wasn't a big deal when I was growing up. In June, my family always headed to Manitoba's immense lake country, where far more exciting things than Father's Day awaited. Sure, we'd make cards or our mom would pick up a gift (usually something jokey, such as a ball cap with a change pouch attached for use at arcades), but the majority of the day was spent at the cottage barbequing and swimming.

By the time my first would-be Father's Day arrived in 2010, we were still within a year of miscarriage, and I hadn't given up hope; but as the second, third, and fourth rolled through, it hurt more and more. Eventually, it got to be too much, and even though I obviously wanted to honor both my own father and my wife's, I asked my family (unsuccessfully) that we not do anything to commemorate the day. Yes, I was lucky at this point to still have both my father and father-in-law in my life, and by right they should have been celebrated, but it was just getting to be too much for me to sit at a brunch while other dads tried to control their munchkins. I suppose I could've reverted to childish ways to *really* make those elder statesmen feel appreciated, but I didn't think an outburst would look good (even if it was just Pancake House we were at).

And here's where things got really weird. In June of 2015, my long-awaited fatherhood was finally imminent (my daughter was born just a couple of weeks later). Yet I couldn't bring myself to celebrate—and we didn't the next year, either. Partly I felt it wasn't right, when so many of my infertile brothers were still suffering; but more personally, Father's Day still felt like a painful reminder that I hadn't done things naturally. It made me feel extremely secondary to the whole process.

My feelings, as you can imagine, aren't unique.

In 2020, a group of males in a men-only infertility group on Facebook shared their sentiments about Father's Day amid responses to a post that simply stated, "Big love and support for anyone struggling today, we're all here for you."

The responses, not surprisingly, were highly charged. One board member openly shared, "I've been crying most of the morning," and a response of, "I have definitely had an emotional weekend too. You're not alone with the tears, bud," followed.

Most of the other comments expressed similar resentment and isolation on the day; but amid the storm, there was one bright ray of light. "Thanks buddy. Great post. Real tough day," one member posted. "We did find out we have an embryo to transfer this morning. 🤞 just gotta keep on trucking. Stay strong my friends."

Messages like these can be a lifeline, but could we be doing more as a society to raise awareness of how the holiday feels to men who are suffering through infertility? Absolutely; and in the eyes of one now-father, we should take our cues from the compassion shown toward all women on Mother's Day.

In 2016, Spencer Blake offered some insight on the subject for *Time* magazine. In an op-ed about Father's Day, Blake reflected on the disparity. "I've noticed lately that there is a lot more awareness for women in general on Mother's Day—single mothers, widows, those who have lost children, those who can't or don't have children. I'm glad to see the growing sentiment of inclusiveness for them on a day that, for many, is absolutely grueling on an emotional level," he stated. "I haven't, however, noticed that there's much emphasis on men of all kinds when it comes to Father's Day."[2]

So how *do* you deal with Father's Day when you're struggling to become a dad? In a post for the Texas Fertility Center, Dr. Erika Munch suggested four paths, including making time for friends and family that doesn't involve children, spending the day with your partner, avoiding kid-laden locations, and being open with your feelings.

Personally, I stand by my original MO—ignore the day. Disconnect from social media, which is filled with smiling dads and their kids, and go camping or on a lengthy nature walk. Spend the day with your partner on the sofa and crank Netflix.

But most importantly, be upfront with your family. While my own pleas may have fallen on deaf ears at times, it is fully within your right to tell your parents or sibling that you need a kid-free day. Make an alternate plan with just your father or father-in-law, such as golfing. Pretty much the best solution, as any would-be mother who feels the sting of being without a child on Mother's Day would say, would be to go wherever kids can't go. Choose the pub instead of Chuck E. Cheese, for example.

Or, if you are like a large part of the infertile crowd, take your dog for a walk and enjoy some time with your fur baby.

CHAPTER 19

Our Furry Children

Time and time again, studies have shown that pets can be miraculous cures for emotional distress or mental turmoil. Whether you're housing a cat, dog, hamster, or iguana, the relative cuteness of the pet and seeing its face when you come home from a long day of work will put a smile on yours ... well, at least until you see what they've been up to all day.

This is especially true among senior citizens. As noted by petsforthe elderly.org, "New research confirms and expands earlier studies indicating a link between pet ownership and a reduced risk of developing heart disease."

But the therapeutic value of animals isn't restricted to seniors, by any stretch. Perhaps unsurprisingly, many couples struggling to conceive have reported finding comfort in their pets—and while a dog won't cure motility issues, it can certainly ease the pain of uncertainty.

Witness what Greg Sdeo said of his dog Lila after she passed. In his blog *A Few Pieces Missing from Normalcy—An Infertile Man's Perspective*, Greg talked about how crucial she had been not only in helping him cope with the childless life that fate had dealt him but in keeping his marriage together.

"Lila was with us during our darkest days, from finding out about my infertility to our journey to parenthood ending," Sdeo wrote. "No matter how dark the day, she always made us smile. She became a part of the family that everyone loved. Her calm demeanor helped my MIL [mother-in-law] overcome her fear of dogs, leading my in-laws to get a dog of their own. If not for her, I am not sure K and I would have made it through infertility and being childless."[1]

Speaking with Sdeo, even after much time had passed since he penned that post, gave me a keen sense of just how special Lila, a retired greyhound they rescued, was to him and his wife. "We had adopted her a few months before we found out about my infertility," Sdeo told me. "In fact, had we been able to have children, chances are we never would have adopted her, which is sad, because she was a great dog who taught us a lot about life. Not so much a particular moment, but everyday life. Later this month it will be a year since she has passed and there isn't a day that goes by that we don't think about her."

Sdeo added that he is not alone in his feelings. He commented, "I have found that the majority of couples that I've connected with that have gone through infertility have pets, even the ones that ended up going on to have children."

I've seen the same myself; the majority of my support group in Winnipeg had a dog, a cat, or another animal. There's a natural transition here; if you cannot parent a child, you'll choose to nurture another being. After all, that instinct doesn't extinguish if you don't get pregnant—in fact, it can grow much stronger.

And let's be honest—some pets are a lot like babies. Though most don't wear diapers (I emphasize *most*), consider the following evidence:

- Often, an owner of a small dog will carry it up and down stairs or even during walks when its legs get tired, much the same way that a parent will trot a child during a long walk or upstairs to bed (and yes, both babes of skin and babes of fur will whine and complain if they don't want to go to bed). There are some owners who prepare for this, additionally, by getting carriers that wrap around your body the same way you would wear them for a human baby. Want something less humiliating (in theory)? There are actually humans that put their dogs or cats in strollers.

- Getting your home pet-ready is similar to baby-proofing. Chances are, if you are bringing home a new puppy, you're going to put away anything that can be destroyed by claws, chewing, or accidents. Also, as YouTube has demonstrated countless times, Christmas trees are just as much in jeopardy with a pet as they are with a child.

- Speaking of accidents, babies will leak out their diapers at the most inopportune time, and even the most loyal and trained pet will occasionally do its dirty work in spots you'd wish it wouldn't. Though their . . . shall we say . . . releases aren't similar, the guilty looks can be. And both child and pet may try to clean up their own mess, with predictable results.

- We all know that parents are suckers for spoiling their babies. You can pretty much put the term *baby* on anything and *some* overeager parent will buy it. Pets? Well they're just as pampered, if not more so: outfits, toys, spa treatments. Need proof? Google *dog psychologist*, *cat cafe*, or *pet spa*.

- Did we get to feedings yet? Training comes in here as well, and no matter how much you keep a pet or baby on schedule, there will be times that they just want to eat. Often, this comes somewhere around 4 a.m., when a parent/owner is deep in a (probably rare) REM cycle. Pets have the perfect way of letting their owners know they're hungry: they'll climb into bed and stand on your stomach, hair, or face, or howl loud enough to wake up the neighborhood. Pets are also quite naive when it comes to hunger, and they're as liable to take food from a stranger as a kid is to willingly accept candy from anyone (though it's near impossible to get a pet to shout "Stranger danger!").

- Their language skills are similar. If you think people become nauseating babblers of a kindergarten level when a newborn is in the room, wait until you see what happens when a new dog or cat arrives. The unintelligible noises that emit from a new pet owner or a friend visiting are enough to make you appreciate the subtle eloquence of a text.

Oh, and then there are pictures. Lots of pictures. The single most annoying thing to an infertile couple is going on Facebook or Instagram and seeing people post pictures of every waking moment of their baby's life. No lie—there are some delusional parents who actually think that other people want to see their baby's poop.

Pet owners can get just as snap-happy. The fur babies are so adorable as they play, sleep, and leave paw prints after walking through water (or worse). And just as parents will dress their kids up in costumes or holiday sweaters, or hire professionals for Christmas cards, so, too, will pet owners.

The therapeutic nature of pets goes well beyond their similarities to babies, though. For a family anxious to celebrate good news, a pet is a welcome change from posting about their BFNs as they struggle with infertility. Blogger Julie Pippert, in an entry titled "Women with Big Dogs (and Infertility)," spoke about her struggles to conceive and how the pending arrival of her chocolate Labrador was generating excitement not only for her and her husband but for her entire relationship circle.

"As we waited for our puppy to reach the magical 'ready to be adopted' age, we shared with family and friends that we'd have a dog soon," she wrote. "We were so happy to have good news to share, about an expected event. Our friends and family were so happy to have good news to express joy over. We were very pleased with ourselves, and everyone relished the break from the 'no news is bad news' phase we'd been loitering in a few years too long."

That feeling of celebration goes beyond the excitement that Pippert describes. For an infertile couple, a pet serves as a fantastic distraction from the root of their frustration, and can help bring them back together during what might otherwise be a very divisive time in their relationship. After all, how can you fight when cute puppy eyes are staring up at you? (Okay, maybe you can, but you feel *really* bad afterward.) Truthfully, there is no better therapy than taking the family dog for a walk or tossing a tennis ball in the backyard.

This certainly was the case in my family.

A couple of years into our fertility struggles, my wife's itch to take care of a being—any being—became too powerful not to scratch. We lightly talked about it for a few weeks before the hunt became real.

One hot summer day, I got a call at my office. My wife had answered an online ad for a mini dachshund. She had already gone down to see the dog once that day but wanted me to come as well after work . . . and bring money. Yep, there was no way we weren't going home without this little guy.

His name was Mercer. He was, we were told, a five-year-old purebred, though we later ID'd him as a dachshund/beagle cross (the nosiest of all pups, I am certain). The previous owners had unsuccessfully tried mating him with a full-size dachshund, but the two dogs never got along—in fact, Mercer had been bitten on the top of the head by the other dog at some point. This was, as far as we knew, his second home, though I suspected there had been more. When we later contacted his veterinarian of record and found that he was actually not on file, we were a bit mystified and ultimately felt sorry for this seventeen-pound (and very overweight) doxie. All we knew was that he had lived with this family in their basement, peeing on pads almost all of his life there. I was suspicious that the aforementioned bite wasn't the only abuse he had suffered.

Within an hour of our seeing him, Mercer was packed into our car and on the way to our house. Because he hadn't been properly taken care of, we knew it was going to be a struggle to train him. The first night, he slept on a chair on the main floor of our two-story home, free from the cat carrier. We let him get acquainted with his new surroundings, especially the backyard, where he could run free.

He was very quiet and didn't do much barking, unusual for a mini dachshund. The first few days were hell, as we tried everything we could think of to get him to eat and avoid co-sleeping. On day three I came home to see my wife victoriously holding out her hand, off of which Mercer was eating wet food. Eventually we got him onto dry kibble instead.

It took a couple of months for him to warm up to me. We'd been told he had issues with men, and it showed. Once he started sleeping in our bed—which we knew from the start was inevitable—he would either bark at me when I tried to come in or purposely lie across my pillow, claiming it as his own. At one point early on I tried to change his name to Messier in recognition of one of my favorite hockey players (and in tribute to his defensive greatness), but it didn't work.

Mercer soon became a fixture in our family. We took him to holiday celebrations (and not shockingly, he loved gefilte fish) and had our parents watch him early on when we went on date nights (before we decided he could be in our house on his own). He came with us on road trips, even across the border to Grand Forks, North Dakota, a popular destination for Winnipeggers. When he needed socialization, he went to dog parks and occasionally off to summer "camp." Oh, and if you're curious, we also took family photos with him. Plenty of family photos.

I wasn't the fondest of him at first, and he felt the same about me;

but as time went on, my fatherly instincts kicked in, and as much as he resisted, we started to do some daddy-doggy bonding—going for walks and drives, playing in the backyard, and singing songs (if howling together counts as singing). Mercer also dutifully fulfilled my very male need to not only care for another being but to push it past its supposed limits. While I stopped short of training him to fetch a beer, I did challenge him to a 5K walk (definitely not easy on such small legs).

Even if Mercer never finished the walk, or fetched me a beer or learned to pee in the toilet, I wouldn't trade any of it. To teach a once-helpless animal the many wonders of the world around him is about as satisfying as life gets, I think.

CHAPTER 20

Adoption and Other Options

Back in the late 1980s and early 1990s, you often ran into kids on the playground who were adopted by their parents. I never thought much about it, although I'm sure those children did.

In fact, while talking about this book with friends of my in-laws during the summer of 2019, I learned that they had adopted both of their children. I was surprised at first, but I soon remembered how commonplace it seemed then, compared to today.

Statistics from the Adoption Network, an agency based in the US, say that 135,000 kids are adopted annually in the States. This seems like a lot, until you consider that there are 310 cities in the States with populations over 100,000. If we played just with those two numbers, that's fewer than 450 adoptions, on average, taking place in those markets each year. And when my wife and I investigated public adoption, we discovered that fewer than fifty adoptions took place through public agencies in Winnipeg in an average year.

Suddenly, the adoption rate doesn't seem that high, does it? It actually has fallen in recent years. As Karla King points out in an article for adoption.org, 1971 saw 90,000 children placed for adoption.[1] That number drastically fell some forty years later: "By 2014, that rate had dropped to 18,000 infants under the age of 2. That means that in all successful births in the United States, adoption rates have fallen from 9% to a mere 1%."

King attributed the swing to a few different factors, among them advances in fertility technology (remember, IVF didn't come along until the 1980s), but also societal changes that made teenage pregnancy less stigmatized (as well as less common) and abortion legal. Still, the United States, according to King's research, has the highest rate of adoption in the world, with 40 percent of adoptees coming out of the foster care system.

Adoption raises many complex emotions and questions. Today, there are several roads you can pursue, but each comes with limitations and trade-offs.

What's interesting is how men and women seemingly view adoption. In its article "Moving from Infertility to Adoption," Canada Adopts! states that "typically, one partner (usually the female, in adoption circles typically known as the 'dragger') will push for adoption, while the other (usually the male, known as the 'draggee') will want to explore other possibilities on the medical front."[2]

I can certainly relate to this; I found the adoption process incredibly nerve-racking when we started looking into it. Amid the aimlessness of our unexplained infertility, though, it seemed like a natural way to take some concrete steps. We had already heard that adoption was a two-to-three-year process at least, so even as we were starting to look at assistive procedures, we were also jockeying for a place in that line.

There are generally three ways one can adopt:

1. Public adoption. The most common method, done through a jurisdiction-run agency or service. In some areas, public adoption involves a child removed from their family for safety reasons as judged by the jurisdiction, and in many

cases, it's a foster-to-adopt process, which can be much more emotionally taxing than a straight adoption.

2. Private adoption. This is through agencies in the more traditional model that most folks are likely familiar with. Though orphanages were never as common as they might seem if you're a Broadway fan (or had to suffer through *Annie* being a musical at your school), private agencies do generally move quicker than public adoption. Depending on where you live, private adoption may happen most often in the case of a mother (and/or father) surrendering her child.

3. International adoption. Because of the prevalence in some countries, international adoption may very well be the one you think of initially; but adopting from jurisdictions outside the US has had significant decreases. In 2018, the *Conversation* reported a major drop in international adoptions, down from circa 46,000 children in 2005 (just about half coming to the US) to 12,000 total in 2015 (5,500 to the States). Changes have come for a variety of reasons, but *Conversation* authors Mark Montgomery and Irene Powell cited a couple of examples. In 2012, Russia closed its doors to foreign adoption to the United States after a two-year-old died after being locked in a car by his new father, while Ethiopia closed its borders in 2013 after a thirteen-year-old girl passed away from hypothermia and malnutrition in the US. Also cited was a drastic reduction in adoptions from China, which decreased by 86 percent from the late 1990s. Still, the option is available in several jurisdictions. It's important to know that in international adoption, the country you are adopting from dictates the rules. In some cases, this means relocating to that country for a period to show that your new child would be coming into a home that retains the country's culture.

———

Partly due to finances, since we knew a big bill was likely in our future as we continued to investigate assistive reproduction, we explored the public route first.

As part of our adoption investigation, we had to attend a seminar where social workers, experienced adoptive parents, and adoptees talked about the process. As we expected, others there were struggling with infertility as well. What we didn't expect was a new mother breast-feeding her three-month-old in the middle of the room. I could feel the eyes of the other attendees on her.

So, back to the dragger versus dragee. By the time the seminar was done, I was feeling more hesitant. One of the adoptive couples was one of those "miracle" families that have a child naturally after adoption. They reflected that, as much as they fought it, they still wanted a biological child after they adopted, and were feeling truly blessed after they were able to conceive. It hit both me and my wife pretty hard, but more so me, if I'm being honest.

The lead presenter chose then, for reasons unknown, to remark that adoption was not a cure for infertility—that you wouldn't be walking "your daughter" down the aisle at her wedding.

I think I actually gasped out loud at that one, and I *know* I became the old man at the typewriter later on, sending off an email to the organizers about her insensitivity.

Still, I was not completely soured on adoption, and I wanted to keep our options open. But the next step was one of the most emotional undertakings I've ever experienced, either alone or with my wife.

One of the unfortunate realities of the adoption process is that you are likely going to be adopting a child with a disability, if not multiple disabilities. These can be physical, mental, or emotional. In the case of our public adoption forms, we had to go through a very extensive list of disabilities and assess what we could reasonably handle under our care. This ranged from needing a wheelchair or other mobility assistance to having attachment disorders or fetal alcohol syndrome.

There is nothing more heart-wrenching than talking about what kind of childhood challenges you would and would not be able to, for lack of a better term, live with. The process is fair, of course—and important—but it's not an easy conversation to have, either with yourself or your partner. Suffice it to say, we went through a lot of Kleenex.

Still, we soldiered through until we were on the list for visitations—i.e., an official visit to our home to check things out to see if we were properly ready to house a child. While adoption can take many years to happen, it can also occur with little more than a moment's notice, so you really do have to be ready.

At this point, though, we decided to walk away from adoption and pursue medical treatments. And one big reason, though I hate to admit it, is that the presenter who offended me was on to something: adoption isn't the cure for infertility. Yes, you have your child, but there's a chance you may still feel your family isn't complete the way you'd want it to be. And to complicate things further, you may feel guilty for feeling this way!

Amy Weber speaks to this. As president of Infertility and Adoption Support, Inc., in St. Louis, she sees commonalities in the emotions her client couples are experiencing. "I don't feel like many people, women especially, ever truly 'get over' their infertility," she says. "In fact, I know many women who are years past the finalization of their child(ren)'s adoptions who still have feelings of sadness when others announce their pregnancy. It's so hard to give up that desire to carry your own child, especially when you go through years of infertility treatments. I think that when a couple chooses to pursue adoption, they are choosing a different path, even though the desire to carry a child is still there, and maybe never truly goes away."

Certainly, that longing is understandable, but ultimately adoption happens for a reason—often, that a family wants to give a child who has been abandoned or removed from his or her surroundings a better chance in life. It's an extraordinarily noble deed, and the families who do this have my deepest respect.

And when I say families, I mean that truly. In contrast to what Canada Adopts! stated, Weber views the male's role in the adoption process as equal. "I don't necessarily think that men are less willing . . . I think people maybe assume this because the women normally drive the adoption process," she said. "However, there's no way that anyone would go through this process if they weren't willing, even if their partner were pushing it."

Other Paths to Parenthood

Of course, adoption is just one of the alternatives to having a child that comes from both parents and occurs through the traditional carrying means, even with ART.

The first is surrogacy. Couples pursuing this route will most often have a healthy egg and sperm from both parents, and use IVF or a similar procedure so that another woman can carry the child to term. Sounds simple and straightforward, right? Unfortunately not.

Many jurisdictions, Canada included, have not fully legalized surrogacy. Here's the explanation, straight from the government itself: "In Canada, it is a crime to pay (in cash, goods, property or services), offer to pay, or advertise to pay a woman to be a surrogate mother."[3] However, government documentation further states, "Although paying a surrogate mother for her carrying of the child is a crime, a surrogate mother may be repaid for out-of-pocket costs directly related to her pregnancy."

And it doesn't get any less complicated in the United States, as "The Sensible Surrogacy Guide" notes: "Surrogacy in the United States remains unregulated at the federal level, with each individual state having its own laws (or not). The individual state laws vary widely even between states that are considered 'surrogacy friendly.'"[4]

Surrogacy friendly? Okay, I'm listening . . .

"For example, some states allow for surrogacy only for heterosexual couples, while others will allow married couples but not singles."

Discrimination lives!

So what do you do if your jurisdiction doesn't allow for surrogacy? Well, if you're likely to click on a Google ad, you may look to Mexico as an option. An ad for Miracle Surrogacy, advertising a $45,000 procedure, appeared at the top of my search engine more than once, emphasizing the legality of the process. "The answer is 100% yes, in that the federal government does not regulate nor prohibit surrogacy," the company says in their FAQ.[5] "In fact, the courts have fully supported the granting of full parental rights to the biological fathers and honoring and enforcing surrogacy contracts." The clinic provides everything you might need, including passports.

As it turns out, international surrogacy, like international adoption, is surprisingly common. "I know a few Canadian couples [who] ended up coming to Ukraine, where we did surrogacy," said one parent I spoke with, who goes by the nickname Lolly.

Lolly is the author of the blog *Special Surrogacy Journey*. Based in the UK, Lolly and her husband ultimately chose their path owing to a special set of obstacles. Because Lolly had a hysterectomy at an early age, their options for ART were limited. Though the couple did contemplate adoption, it simply wasn't in the cards.

"It's funny, because I was always one of those people who would say 'why don't people just adopt?'" says Lolly. "My brother was adopted, so I understood very well how much love was there, and how genetic makeup made zero difference. However, it was the process for adoption in my country that was so off-putting. Numerous times I have come across adoption boards and councils withholding all the information which is within the intended parents' and child's interests to ensure a speedy adoption process. This, plus the excessive interview process, was so overwhelming. Why is it fair some people can just have a child, whereas others have to lay their heart and soul bare to even be considered?"

Lolly adds that once they knew surrogacy would be their only path, her husband was completely on board with the process, even though restrictions meant they would have to leave the country to do it. "Surrogacy takes a massive leap of faith," she admits. "It took some time for us both to come round to the idea of international surrogacy. But we both saw it as our only hope, so we got on board."

The other option is equally heart-wrenching: donation, be it egg, sperm, or even embryo. Sperm donation, as it turns out, is becoming a more common process. According to statistics revealed by Ashley Fetters in her article for the *Atlantic* titled "The Overlooked Emotions of Sperm Donation," somewhere from thirty thousand to sixty thousand babies born in the US annually are conceived through donated sperm—roughly 1 percent of total births.

Fetters's article looks deeply into the emotionality of the process. For a male spouse or partner, it's often a pain point, which she discussed with Aaron Buckwalter, a marriage and family therapist in California. Buckwalter noted that the male partner (as opposed to a female considering egg donation) can be "much more attached to these ideas of ownership and [the child being] *'mine,'* and much more tied to the genetic connection in terms of what it means psychologically or emotionally.

"These men are often grappling with the question, *Is this my child or someone else's?* That's a tough struggle for a lot of guys when I meet them," Buckwalter adds.

There are, of course, two other parts of the equation within a donation, one of which is the man who has offered his sperm. While the opening scene of *The Big Bang Theory* series, which saw Leonard and Sheldon going to produce in exchange for some needed cash, makes donating seem easy, it's rarely true. Witness Ian's story. In a piece for the Victorian Assisted Reproductive Treatment Authority's website, the seven-time donation father talked about his feelings now, as a married dad of two. "At times I feel quite anguished that I have seven other children somewhere in the world who carry a part of me and my genetic and family background but over whose lives I have no direct influence at all. I wonder if they are alive, if they are healthy, happy, well cared for and loved. I hope that they are, but all I can do is hope," he wrote. "One day I may meet some of them—maybe all. Who knows? Or maybe I will meet none and will forever wonder about them. It seems to me that the process of being a sperm donor is somewhat akin to giving a child up for adoption, with all of these wonderings and anxieties left with the relinquishing parent, or in my case, the donor."

Last, but most important, of course, are the feelings of the children themselves—a key factor if you're considering the donation route. Meet Courtney McKinney, the child of a sperm donor. McKinney talked about the struggle of not knowing both parents in an op-ed for the *Los Angeles Times*.

"That lack of consideration is something I feel the consequences of every time I'm asked where my parents live, every time a doctor wants my family medical history, every time I'm confronted with being biracial (my mom is black but there were no black sperm donors at her cryobank in '89) and every time I wonder what attributes of mine come from this anonymous man," McKinney wrote.

Of course, these are just the ways to have a kid outside of natural conception or ART procedures. There is also the other option, one that can be much scarier to wrestle with: not having kids at all.

CHAPTER 21

Coping with Childlessness

Throughout my infertility journey, there was one very tough question always lingering in the back of my mind: "What if it doesn't happen?"

What if the treatments don't work? What if our adoption path falls through? What if we can't find a surrogate?

Too many uncertainties, too many possibilities, too much chance that we'd ultimately have to move on with our lives as a couple and not the full family we hoped to have in our three-bedroom, two-story, one-and-a-half-bath house. At one point we even said that if we weren't successful, we'd give up our "family home" and go back to condo life. After all, without kids, who needs a big backyard for a swing set, or a place to camp out a couple of nights every summer? It would just be too much space for us to look out on and think of what could have been.

This fear was not unfounded. Most IVF treatment centers (still) have fairly long odds, under 50 percent. One in two is good odds when you're playing scratch-offs for a few bucks, but this is just a wee bit higher stakes.

It's not surprising that some couples who go through it set a limit on how many times they'll try. Every round does a number on the female

137

body—more drugs, more injections, another emotional roller coaster. Many couples will look at alternative means, such as adoption or surrogacy, but those are fraught with their own risks of failure. And of course, it all costs money—something of which most folks don't have an endless supply.

While in our support group, we saw this take place firsthand. Some couples either stopped trying to have kids or left, while the others, whom we had bonded with, began having success. Though we no longer attended the support meetings after having our daughter, we kept tabs on the others as best we could, including those who had gone through so much without the same reward.

There's no question—we all could have done more to support our brothers and sisters in arms and needles, but at the same time, we were starting to become those parents-to-be that infertile people sometimes distanced themselves from. Yes, our journeys had been longer and harder than most, and we'd all earned our stripes, but we understood why we didn't hear from those couples anymore. Occasionally we would ask around the room or in Facebook groups if anyone had heard anything, but more often than not, no one had a read.

It's here that a challenge arises: what care is provided for a couple who depart from the infertility grid?

"When a couple is identified as having an infertility challenge, they are then shunted into the infertility space, they are there for treatment, whether it's a month or ten years or whatever it might be, and within that time period, there are emotional struggles. That's where our world has been dealing with men and their experiences," says Dr. Eleanor Stevenson, "but I think when you have some of those dysfunctional adaptations that result from not being successful, they very often happen as a result of not trying to continue treatment, and that's where we lose touch with our patients. We don't follow them. If they're not part of the infertility care system, they're lost to us."

And post-care cessation is the true closing of a door, as Dr. Stevenson suggests. "I don't know of any work that has looked at the post-discharge or post-discontinuation care plan," she continues. "I'm not sure what kind of resources or evaluation is given to patients at the time they decide to discontinue treatment. The number one reason people discontinue treatment is emotional. It's not because they run out of money, it's not because they're told there are no more options—it's the emotional distress."

In the years since those group days, I've spoken with some childless individuals and couples. It's never been easy. Some put their energy into nieces and nephews, others into their pets; others just enjoy each other's company and live a life of adventure and travel. No one can judge how they choose to move on.

What we do know about the pain of childlessness, again, is largely focused on women desiring to be mothers. There hasn't been that much research into how it affects the male psyche. Dr. Robin Hadley, himself childless, was one of the first to approach the subject directly. In 2018, he spoke to the *Guardian* about his recently released study.[1]

"I found," he told writer Bibi Lynch, herself also childless, "there was little difference in the desire to become a parent between female and male childless individuals. But that study also indicated that for some male participants, not becoming a parent had a greater negative effect. That's because there are no narratives around childlessness for men."

Lynch also spoke with a childless male by the name of Kelsey. Circumstance hadn't allowed him to have a kid at the time of publication (he was forty-three and single), and he felt deep regret and emptiness.

"I was really desperate for children, even in my early twenties. Because of my own childhood, I wanted a son. I never thought about having a daughter. I knew I couldn't change my childhood, which was traumatic, but I thought I could give a child—a boy—the childhood I didn't have. I thought I'd be a really good dad," Kelsey told Lynch. "The first time it hit me that I might not have children was when I turned thirty. I was upset and talking to my friends and they said, 'It will happen. You'll see.' But I had a feeling it wouldn't. Then I hit forty and another low: a feeling of, it's really not going to happen now."

Here's the really interesting part of Lynch's story, and in turn Dr. Hadley's research: men outnumber women in childlessness. Consider this 2010 report by Statistics Netherlands:

> *The percentage of men without children has increased in successive generations. One in six men born shortly after World War II does not have any children, compared with one in four born in the period 1960–1964.*
>
> *Relatively fewer women than men are childless. One in five women born in the period 1960–1964 do not have any children. The number of childless women also increased by less. One reason for the higher childlessness among men is that more men remain single.[2]*

The immediate conclusion is that women will resort more often to being a single mom by choice than dads who would try the same thing. Perhaps men are more willing to face a life of solitude, or we simply realize there are some things we just can't do alone.

Whichever the case may be, childlessness is a distinct possibility that every infertile person faces, and no matter how much you try to brush it off, it hurts. Bad.

CHAPTER 22

Speaking Out

Mike Heller has a very different job from most of us.

You see, Mike Heller is a TV writer. As he explained to me, TV writers do exactly what you'd suspect they do—channel their own toils and tribulations into story lines for the shows we all love.

"As a writer, I tend to be more open about things in general. We tend to mine our own lives, and have practice being vulnerable," he said.

What separates Heller is that he took his struggle beyond the writer's room and into the public eye. In March 2020, he penned a blog post for RESOLVE, one of the leading US nonprofits for infertility awareness and support. He described his new, responsible, heroic role as The Injector. Though the name sounds more like a diabolical villain than a hero, his nom de plume was certainly heroic, earned for plunging a needle into his wife every evening as part of her drug protocol.

"In the same half-light each night," Heller wrote in his blog, "I'd eye my wife's stomach, looking for the perfect spot to inject. I'd bend down with quiet focus, keeping the pen as level as possible before inserting it into my wife's abdomen. Then I'd push the cocktail of Follistim and Menopur with my thumb as hard as humanly possible to ensure she got every last drop. And, finally, gingerly, I'd pull it back out. That's it. End of job."

Like any good superhero, The Injector perfected his craft. Batman knew when to throw a bat-a-rang; Heller's timing was similarly impeccable. "It seems simple, but there was an art to it. And I became obsessed with getting it right," Heller continued. "Somehow, I thought, if I executed this perfectly, it would make the difference. If I could make a clean injection, with no bleeding or bruising, the meds would work better than they normally do, and she would get pregnant."

Heller's piece was certainly gutsy. Readers loved his unique take on how he could best contribute to his family's pursuit of a child.

"It was my first go in terms of posts. I hadn't written any articles or blogs," he said. "I have written a half-hour TV show that I have which I'm going to tweak and send around, it's always in the back of my head, but The Injector is really the first.

"The opportunity came my way. My wife came to me and said, 'You should do this!' and I said 'okay.' I wasn't nervous about it. I was sort of excited to share, especially because this is something that I love to talk about. I feel like it's important to talk about, and even in writing my half-hour pilot, my mission statement was that people should be talking about it."

The need that Heller identified came from his own experience of feeling like he "was on a desert island," he said. It's a common refrain among men in the infertility community.

"When we initially went through it, especially at the beginning, we felt like we were so alone in it, and the only people going through it, when that's not even close to being true. So many are going through it and not talking about it. I think it's important just to stay connected and feel like we're not alone."

Getting any sort of voice behind the cause—whether in writing, interviews, or public speaking—is tough as hell. But in the aftermath, you feel incredible.

I won't lie—that first interview was tough. Even with the cloak of anonymity, I was a bundle of nerves. I stumbled, I *umm*ed and *like*d and *you know*ed my way through, but I came out feeling as if a huge weight had been lifted off my shoulders. I've always been one to put myself out there. It's part of why I got into journalism—I have this thing for publicity. I don't chronicle my whole life on social media or anything, but I'm certainly not afraid to share an opinion or be the spokesperson for a cause.

In the days and weeks after "Greg" made his radio broadcast debut, my doubt and fear were quickly replaced by a feeling of responsibility— that if no one else was going to speak, then I had to. And it evolved very rapidly.

Soon after the initial radio broadcast came Canadian Infertility Awareness Week. Annually in April or May, representatives from across the country speak at events and to media about the invisible crisis. I found myself on the steps of my provincial legislature providing the first of what would become frequent public addresses about infertility. I prepped alongside others who were going to be available to talk with the press, but I was the only man. While I wasn't completely conscious of when the media had arrived on scene, I knew the crowd would go well beyond the typical support group members and parents.

I was nervous as I pulled my infertility T-shirt over my long-sleeve and practiced the few bullet points I had prepared. Thankfully, I'd be speaking to plenty of people in the same situation I was. It was the next step in opening up the dialogue. Talking for taped camera interviews that day was just as nerve-racking, yet I was going to be fairly straight-forward with it. Just repeat what you said on the steps, I told myself, and it will go okay.

A couple of days later I was invited to my local CTV studio, along-side a female member of our support group, for a live interview on their morning show. Live interviews are about the scariest situation ever, par-ticularly on TV. In radio, you have a safety net, not just in no one being able to see you, but most microphones have a handy "cough" button you can hit to temporarily mute your mic. On television, there's no such thing. You stumble over words; you show all your weird tics; or, at absolute worst, an inelegant word is picked up by the censors. Either way, you can pooch future opportunities with a single slip.

One trick that I've learned over the years is to not focus on the camera lights around you, and to make the interview into a conversation. The best broadcasters and journalists will lead in this manner, but it's just as important for you to follow suit and concentrate only on them, not on the cameras or producers or studio audience.

Of course, you're also running against the clock, since segments can be three minutes long or even less, and when you're trying to convey a story as personal as infertility, it's not much. The key is pacing yourself and practicing. I've coached many officials and business owners in this, and I still make a habit of rewatching every interview I do to see where my quirks are.

The same goes if you're starting to write your story or an advice blog, as many people are now doing. Yes, there is the potential for an endless amount of space on a webpage, but readers will want something more straightforward with some color added in.

It quickly became clear that most people had never seen a man speaking out about infertility. After that CTV interview I did several others, culminating with an interview about Movember, wherein I described how my well-being was tied directly to my infertility struggle.

Then along came TED—or, more specifically, TEDx.

I had long been fascinated by TED. If you haven't listened to or watched a TED Talk, I highly recommend you do so. Some are funny, some are deeply serious, but they're always enlightening. Some of the greatest minds of this era have given TED Talks, including heroes of mine like the journalist A. J. Jacobs.

At first, I thought I had a cool story to talk about in how I turned childhood passions for wrestling and trading cards into a career high-lighted by working for Topps on their WWE products. Boy, would that address have been easy to give.

I studied so many TED and TEDx Talks in prep for my delivery, and was pleasantly surprised to find that other men were using the platform to discuss infertility. Among them was Alon Neuman at TEDx Jerusalem, who in 2015 gave a talk entitled "IVF, Fertility Treatments & Men: A Puz-zling Proposition." Just over a minute in, Neuman gave this introduction:

> *Many have researched the wonders and technicalities of birth,*
> *and there is endless literature on the subject, but I thought it*
> *would be interesting to share with you the patient's perspective—*
> *or, to be more precise, the perspective of a puzzled male.*

Neuman's talk was inspirational for me, and helped me swallow any fear I had of putting myself out there on the dreaded Internet. In the years since, I've seen so many more men share their experiences, in one form or another, without anonymity. It's astounding how quickly the community, nearly nonexistent when I did that first interview, has grown, particularly when you consider that the role models most of us look to—athletes and entertainers—haven't been as vocal as we might hope. But even that is changing. In the next chapter, we'll see who's shed-ding new light on a conversation still shrouded in darkness.

CHAPTER 23

The Effects of Pop Culture

The funny thing about infertility is that when you're in it, there is this overwhelming feeling that everyone around you either has new kids, is pregnant, or will soon be. Babies are suddenly everywhere.

As a guy, it's easier to escape this to an extent, since you can't pick a father-to-be out of a lineup; but women? Yes, as shocking as this sounds, guys look at women. Married, single, friends with benefits . . . no matter the situation, we look.

And when you're in an infertile state, you see the pregnancy bumps.

What hasn't helped is the deluge of pop culture and the explosion of TV shows to fill the suddenly endless channels and streaming services— both real-life and scripted stories. And naturally, the shiny, happy pregnancy shows far outnumber the infertility stories.

During the first round of infertility, there were two very different reality shows that factored prominently into our lives, one focused on pregnancy and one not so pregnant.

The show that appealed to me more was *Giuliana & Bill*, a series about the then-host of *E! News* and her husband, the winner of *The Apprentice*.

Giuliana and Bill Rancic were the rare couple who went public early on about their infertility. Even though much of the show focused on Giuliana's feelings—as it was female factor infertility—there was a comfort in watching them go through something so similar to what we were experiencing.

This was in stark contrast to another show that was beamed into my home (and many, many others). For whatever reason, some infertile folks found MTV's *Teen Mom* (and *16 and Pregnant*, its "sister" show) strangely compelling. I didn't get it, until I started curiously googling.

Witness a thread that came up in the r/infertility channel on Reddit. One poster, KittyL0ver, was pretty succinct in her assessment. "I started watching it as a guilty pleasure, and for whatever reason, still watch occasionally," she said.

Others weren't quite as forgiving. "I don't have time for TV like that anymore," said original poster (or OP, for all you hepcats) Semirelatednonsense, "nor would I torture myself by watching irresponsible dumb asses get knocked up while I'm over here peeing on sticks every other day and waking up at 5:30 on weekends to take my stupid bbt knowing it's going to be the same as it was the day before. Not to mention I don't even remember how to use a tampon anymore it's been so long."

But there was another insight among these contrasting opinions, one that summed up, I think more accurately, how many women felt: shows like *Teen Mom* are an escape. Reddit user Lohryn explained it succinctly. "I still watch and love *Teen Mom*. It's hard sometimes. But then I think—if I had to switch places with them to get children, would I? Heck no! The same is true with people in my personal life. It sucks and is so painful, but I'll take infertility and no babies with my husband and my life over any other circumstance."

I think Lohryn, intentionally or otherwise, has hit on one of the best ways to deal with infertility—escape it! This is important for both you and your partner, individually and together. Finding anything, and I mean *anything*, that can get your mind off it is the healthiest thing you can do. Yes, trash TV, social media, and the like aren't exactly marathon training, but when you're trying so hard to make something "right," burying yourself in your own head won't help, either.

Celebrity gossip is one tried-and-true way to distract ourselves. Tabloid magazines like *Hello!* and the *National Enquirer* exist for a reason, as do shows like *Entertainment Tonight* and *TMZ*. But here's the interesting thing about celebs—they also have the immense power to influence our lives, for better or for worse.

In the infertile world, there have been many, *many* female stars who have shared their stories, including Amy Schumer and Gabrielle Union. Men, however, have very few examples, and most often speak in tandem with their partner. Chrissy Teigen, for example, has been more open than her beau, John Legend, and Michelle Obama opened up about her IVF, while Barack has been silent.

This begs the question, then—if there were more high-profile men who spoke up, would it help? I think so, even if what it does is simply throw more light on the struggle. This is what Mike Heller, a fertility patient, sees as the biggest benefit, even if these people's lives seem out of reach in other ways.

"We know that it exists in the world, and some people go through it," says Heller. "Some female celebrities speaking out about it is nice, and it helps start the conversation. I just think that no one in our real lives were talking about it. It's a separate category, at least for me. They're celebrities, in a different category, and almost not real."

So how much do men really speak out? Well, Legend is inarguably the most prominent name to bring a male voice to infertility. In 2017, Legend talked about his and Teigen's journey to *Cosmopolitan* reporter Mia Lardiere, saying, "I think it's especially difficult when you can't conceive naturally. You want to feel like everything's working properly and want everything to be perfect, but sometimes it's not. I wouldn't say we can't conceive naturally, but I would say that it's enough of a challenge where it felt like we needed help."

Legend and Teigen had their first child, a daughter, Luna, via IVF, as well as a subsequent son, Miles.

Other names are a bit more niche, but have given light just as openly. In April 2019, WWE superstar Tommaso Ciampa told his story through one of the company's YouTube accounts. Amid a video that detailed his surgery to repair a broken neck, Ciampa was shown holding his baby girl, Willow.

"My wife and I wanted to have a child for a long time, and we couldn't. We finally discovered the only option we had was in vitro," Ciampa said in the video. "In vitro was a lot more than we ever thought as far as, not just financially, but what a process emotionally. Miscarriages . . . take a toll, especially on the mom. It's the hardest thing we ever went through, for sure."

And before either Legend or Ciampa, Robert Mathis was thrust into a spotlight. In 2014, the now-retired linebacker, once of the Indianap-olis Colts, was suspended from NFL play due to banned substances in his bloodstream. The source, however, wasn't your usual performance-enhancing drug; it was Clomid. His wife had been on Clomid for their twin boys earlier, and her condition had deteriorated in the years follow-ing. "But in the end, with this child, with baby Brielle, the doctor said she couldn't take anything, or it would be harmful to her, maybe even cause death. So I got checked out, and the doctor in Atlanta prescribed it for me," Mathis told *Esquire*.

The Clomid prescription was in part to help Mathis's low sperm count. "To keep weight on and my performance and whatnot and the reason we weren't able to conceive. I got a blood test, and the results from that—it was low sperm count, low [testosterone], and they just pre-scribed that to help me with the baby."

These real-life examples, however, are perhaps lesser known than the stories we see on broadcast television. Shows like *The Big Bang Theory*,

This Is Us, *Life in Pieces*, *How I Met Your Mother*, *Friends*, and countless others have had infertility story lines as far back as the '90s. On the silver screen, infertility has largely been part of a larger story, such as in the Disney/Pixar animated flick *Up* and the Steve Martin/Jack Black/Luke Wilson comedy *The Big Year*. In 2018, it finally got the full Hollywood treatment in the Paul Giamatti film *Private Life*.

In fact, a hot topic in infertility circles has been the accuracy of the accounts in movies and on TV. Some have been celebrated, while others have been decried. Whether infertility becomes a vehicle for a particular character or drives a series or multi-episode arc, each case has its backers and its detractors.

If there is any voice of authority on the subject, it's Heller, now a father of three. He's a writer for various television shows and, at least as of mid-2020, had been working on an infertility-centric script. He feels the work so far has been strong, but there's plenty more to be done, both for men and women.

"Is it accurate? Yes, only because everyone's experience is different and everyone reacts to it in different ways. I almost feel like, who am I to say it's not right? It's not my experience, but some of it is similar. I'm reluctant to push a judgement call," Heller says. "What I'm really looking for, and what I'm writing, is 'let's show everyone the nitty gritty, show the injections and the hard conversations. There's a lot of good, wide-ranging portrayals out there. I think it's all good. I don't think a show has gone full-bore, deep into it. The emotional side? Yes. A lot of shows are getting into the emotional side, but the physicality . . . I don't know. I think there's a lot more to be mined, but all these portrayals are good for the conversation and lifting the taboo."

Another writer, Josh Huber, has a different perspective on the story lines that come across the airwaves. "On TV, it's always this B story that the couple is working on, and more often than not, it's this funny thing that happened. It's this X-rated thing you're talking about, so writers go, 'We can make jokes about this.' It's low-hanging fruit."

Huber's perspective comes from an interesting place. Huber, an infertility patient who now has a daughter, wrote and directed the movie *Making Babies*, which showcased the struggle of a couple to conceive. The movie was semiautobiographical; Huber says he wanted a way to tell friends about the journey he and his wife went on.

"A lot of the people that we tried to talk to about the infertility process . . . you could tell they were interested to know, but they didn't want to ask because it's a private thing," he explains. "People were interested [in the movie], they found it kind of funny and they empathized. For movie purposes, you want characters who want something. So I took some of the instances of what we went through and heightened it.

"I thought it was a topic a lot of people didn't know about. It was something I did know a lot about, and I wasn't scared to show it as it was."

In fact, Huber went to great lengths to illustrate just how much infertility impacts the overall process of becoming a parent, which, in theory, should be a lot more enjoyable.

"It's a weird thing to go through. It's a process," he says. "You're told that having kids is supposed to be this fun thing and then it becomes this science experiment."

Even as he told his own story, however, Huber admits to a touch of Hollywood exaggeration. "There is an aspect I had to heighten a little bit."

What's interesting about Huber's project is that, while as a male he was able to write about the guy's side fairly smoothly, he admits that he dedicated more time to talking about the female side of infertility, in large part because there is more of a story to tell from the female side. "If you're thinking about this as a writer, you're going to think, 'Let's go as the woman,' because her want is going to be bigger. It really does rest on her a lot," he says. "If they don't get pregnant, she can't help but think, 'I'm broken. This is my fault.' We say it in the movie—as men, all you have to do is jerk off into a jar. A guy has to take that and that's all he has to do. That's it though? He doesn't have to take shots, change his life that much. [As a guy] you're really this bump on a log. You're kind of reduced to donor status. You're this masturbating idiot, which is this weird place to be."

Still, it was important for Huber to portray the male partner in a particular light—to go against the stereotype of an infertile man, to the extent that one exists. "We cast Steve Howey in that role—somebody that's not a wimp. Steve's a huge dude. He's somebody that's 'masculine,'" he says. "The trope is the guy would be this pencil-necked little male that couldn't get it there. I wanted to show that this happens to all different ranges of people."

In writing the script, Huber admits that there is the Hollywood happy ending to *Making Babies*, one that he feels fortunate enough to say was also the end to his journey. He feels, though, that the pain of not succeeding isn't shown often enough. "Not to have a spoiler alert, but they [the main characters] end up getting pregnant. It doesn't always work that way, and there are a lot of stories where it's a bummer," he says. "There are people who worked on the movie or in my life that I'm either pretty sure they used infertility treatments or they tell me outright that they did; and there's a real sad side to all of this that needs to be broached a little bit more. There's a side that isn't happy endings—it doesn't always work. That's tough."

CHAPTER 24

Dad Eyes

At a certain point in life, some women will develop what's commonly called "Mom Eyes."

Mom Eyes see everything small as being cute and cuddly and gush-worthy, particularly little shoes, or "booties." It goes hand in hand with the maternal instinct—once you have (or are expecting) a tiny baby who you think is the cutest little thing, then everything that accompanies her is also the cutest little thing. Put it this way: if you can look at a baby's poop and say, "Aww, look at that little poopie woopie," you officially have Mom Eyes.

This, unfortunately, is where the paradigm shift comes in. Whereas most women might ooh and ahh over a little onesie or bib, a woman struggling with infertility will shy away from them. This is why it's vital to be considerate of feelings when it comes to celebrations such as baby showers and first birthdays. For a friend or relative who's struggling, the celebratory atmosphere can stir up all sorts of negative vibes, discomfort, and all-out sadness.

This is one of the times when men clearly have it easier than women. When a guy is about to become a dad, there isn't a party where the boys get together and give him small baseball caps and action figures to decorate the baby's room with. We aren't programmed to do that. We celebrate things by high-fiving (or at least we did, pre-Covid). We also don't coo over small things, generally. We might look at a shop and say, "Hey, that miniature jersey would look good on my baby" or see a Happy Meal with a toy we want . . . for our kid . . . but that's about the extent of it, at least on the surface.

The truth is that "Dad Eyes" are a thing, too, but for guys it's more experiential—watching a baby take its first steps, playing catch in the backyard, sitting in the room next door while Mom scolds the kid for the first time for staying out past curfew (and secretly saying "way to go" in our heads). Of course, women are all about the experiential, too, but with guys it's more concentrated because it's often the only lens through which we visualize parenthood before it happens. We don't care about baby shoes. Baby shoes are inevitably kicked off, so we don't go gaga over them (pun not intended).

And this is where infertile men suffer compared to "successful" dads. With women, the safeguard, as noted above, is to be cautious about invites to baby-centric events. For guys, the danger zone is in discussion. Friends' kids' activities are virtually impossible to hear about. Karate lessons? No thanks. Taking your kid to his first baseball game? Lovely; the infertile man will stay in the "no-children-allowed" bar or lounge. Seeing your kid as the lead in the school play? Yeah, that's quite all right; the would-be dad will stick to other forms of entertainment to witness bad acting.

So from the start, male infertility can become isolating. Why? Because there are generally four topics that are discussed among males:

1. Sports or entertainment
2. Home renovations
3. Jobs and financials
4. Things our kids do

Now, guys will generally respect when one of their bros is having issues in one of these four areas. If one of the crew, for example, just lost his job or got beat up on the stock market, then they skip the money or job talk. But once you have too many danger zones, the conversation quickly becomes limited. Contrary to popular belief, guys do talk; it's just that a lot of our conversation is very superficial, rather than heart-to-heart.

Now try to introduce a topic that's already so hard to discuss: infertility.

What you won't see in the above list is a lot of feelings. Sure, a guy may question why one loves the Cleveland Browns despite them looking more like the Bad News Bears than a professional team, but ultimately it doesn't go much further. Even the least performatively masculine guy will have trouble talking—much less hearing—about infertility, and the effect it's having on a friend. Guys will show support in quick fashion, and just as quickly shift the conversation to one of the guy safety zones. If they're attentive, they'll avoid talking about their own kids—which is a kind gesture, but not ultimately the connection you might be looking for.

Luckily, times are changing, and there are more outlets today than I could have dreamed of just a decade ago. We'll look at some of them in the chapters to come.

CHAPTER 25

Seeking Kinship (aka Dude, Where's My Infertile Tribe?)

One of the hardest parts of being a male suffering from infertility is finding other men in the same boat.

In a very informal, show-of-hands survey I took during my TEDx Winnipeg Talk in 2017, I asked the audience how many of them knew a woman experiencing infertility. Not surprisingly, the hands shot up. When I asked about men, there were exponentially fewer.

Even in their healthiest times, men have trouble talking about their feelings. Just how bad we are, though, may surprise you. In August 2019, allwomenstalk.com published an article by one Samantha Philips on the subject, and the scribe came up with no fewer than fifteen reasons why guys don't chatter about what's going on inside.[1]

Fifteen? Are we really that bad? Apparently so.

Philips pointed to several reasons, including the male propensity to favor action over words and the avoidance of self-reflection, along with common stereotypes about machoism and societal conditioning, and, perhaps most damning, "they don't know how."

Rather than question the validity of her arguments, though you could, I think our time would be better spent examining the deeper truth behind them. We can come up with all the excuses in the world, but it won't help us change the dynamic—which is hurting men as much as women.

First, you have to account for relativism—comparing men to women. And yes, to a certain extent this is an obvious thing, but what would anything in this world be without a study to validate what we already know?

First, to nonverbal communication. *Scientific American* reported the results of a study conducted by McDuff, Kodra, Kaliouby, and LaFrance in 2017, seeking to find which sex was more expressive in their facial language. These researchers gauged the reactions of two thousand men and women to a series of advertisements. Using a facial coding system (likely not HTML), they registered how men and women reacted differently to what they were seeing. Their base conclusion, as documented by *SA* scribe Cindi May, was as follows:

> *In some ways, the results from this study confirm previous findings of greater emotional expressiveness for women. Women did smile more often than men in response to the ads, and their smiles were longer in duration. They also engaged in more inner brow raises, though the duration of these brow raises did not differ from that of men. These data not only align with the belief that women are more likely than men to display emotion, but also suggest that this tendency extends to negative as well as positive emotions, as inner brow raises are thought to be reflective of states of fear and sadness.*[2]

What followed was something exceedingly interesting:

> *Women were not universally more expressive than men, as men were more likely to demonstrate anger-based facial behaviors*

than women. Men showed more brow furrowing than women,
and their brow furrows were longer than those of women as well.
In addition, lip corner depressors were significantly longer in
men than in women.

So men, despite our alleged emotional flatness, actually do beat women at getting angry. Point—Team XY!

Now for the actual conversation.

A few studies have been conducted that clearly show women speak more than men. An article on the subject from cheatsheet.com shared that women say twenty thousand words per day, while men orate less than half that amount (seven thousand, unless you're an egoist and love hearing yourself talk).[3] Females also speak earlier on in their lives than males and form more complex sentences earlier. I mean . . . that's logical, right? Boys have often been heard saying, "I want chocolate," clearly conveying the message without needing to say, "instead of brussels sprouts!" I like to think it's just that we're more efficient.

So what causes this? Philips wasn't off the mark completely with her chemically based claim about neuroscience (item number one on her list), but it's that darn chromosome that actually makes all the difference in the world. As the cheatsheet.com article describes, "the presence of more testosterone in the male body and brain dampens the need to become a chatty Cathy—hence the reason the term is coined after a woman in the first place."

Good one, cheatsheet.com.

So if you're a woman trying to get a man to open up about infertility woes, you're up against science; and unfortunately, there isn't a single answer of how to defeat it.

In order for a man to be comfortable, he has to truly feel like he's in a safe place, and unfortunately, that may not always be in front of his female companion. Yes, we understand this can be extremely frustrating, but it's so hard to be vulnerable in front of our partners—that is deep in the wiring, too.

So where can men turn? Other men would be the obvious answer, but this doesn't always happen, either.

Circa 2013, my wife and I joined a local support group conducted by the Infertility Awareness Association of Canada (now Fertility Matters Canada). Understandably, she wanted me to go with her, and equally understandably, my question was, "Will other guys be there?"

After going to the first session alone, my wife used her considerable powers of persuasion to get the organizers to set up a session where the women, who had for the most part attended solo, were encouraged to bring their male partners along. Voilà—a couples therapy session.

Well, sort of.

The men may have been there in body, but what about mind and spirit? None of the men spoke that night without prompting; but hey, progress, right?

In subsequent months, men continued to attend, albeit in dwindling numbers, but the silence was still deafening. More often than not, it was the woman giving the update on their situation. I was becoming more comfortable in my infertile skin, but I was clearly more the exception than the norm.

Part of this, admittedly, came from my personal preference for talking to women. For reasons that seemingly go against the norm, I found it reasonably easy to chat in these group settings. Nor, by the way, am I alone in this preference. Witness this testimonial from Anny Kuo. By day, she's a marketing and communications guru. By night, she's an ambassador for RESOLVE and leads support groups for couples and individuals suffering from infertility in the Seattle area. She was also an infertility patient herself.

"I've been in a waiting room to see my doctor and had a very chatty man make small talk while he and his wife were waiting for their appointment, proactively offering that he was on Clomid," Kuo says as she discusses men talking about infertility struggles. "I've received emails from men who are reaching out on behalf of them and their wives to attend support groups. They're looking for something they can do, whether their wives are putting them up to it or they themselves are reaching out, recognizing that they need community support."

So let's add this caveat: not every male will restrict themselves to only wanting to talk to other males; still, there's no situation that one would want more than to talk guy to guy about the struggles. I certainly wish I'd had the outlet as I sat in those support meetings, but what wasn't available to me, or to other males in the room, was a group just for us. Without an outlet to talk among men only, we were more honorary members of the group than full participants. We showed up and supported our partners as they talked, but that was about it.

At one point, I came up with the idea of a pub night. Pool, drinks, and wings are usually enough to grease the wheels for guys, but there was a catch—I was dependent on the female partners telling their men about the event after mentioning it in our Facebook group. I'm sure the message was relayed, but there was little interest expressed overall. My attempt to find other men to share my grief with had all but failed.

I continued going to the group meetings with my wife, and when a social event was folded in, more men did come; but I was still having trouble going deeper with any of them. Thank God the landscape has changed so radically in recent years.

So earlier, we established that men, generally, are limited in what they will talk about with other men. Think sports or home renovation projects (aka the honey-do list). Broaching an incredibly personal topic in casual conversation is not easy, and to be fair, if your friends haven't gone through a similar experience, it's hard for them to relate.

But what about men who have been specifically struggling with infertility? Surely, in the common bond, they would welcome some sort of therapeutic discussion?

Unfortunately, it still doesn't flow easily. In fact, you're more likely to see Clint Eastwood break into song mid-shoot-'em-up movie than to see two men who are struggling to conceive discuss it over beers. They *may* touch on what their partners are going through, but they won't delve deeply into each other's emotional well-being like most women will.

I'm guilty of it myself. There were times, at the peak of our struggle, that several infertile couples would get together for dinner. While the women would gather and talk about progress and procedures, the male conversation was just that—male. Hockey was big, as was work.

So it's understandable that men aren't particularly inclined to seek out support groups. The infertility support groups that exist are overwhelmingly attended by women, usually solo. The occasional husband will appear, clearly comfortable enough in his skin to discuss the subject, but he's the exception.

What we can now say is that unless it is a small, one-on-one situation, guys talking with guys (or women, for that matter) becomes a big dilemma. Trying to talk about anything beyond what's on TV or the food in front of them can be difficult.

The deficit of options for guys to talk to guys isn't limited to the realm of infertility. Amy Klein, a journalist who penned the *Motherlode* blog for the *New York Times* and authored *The Trying Game: Get Through Fertility Treatment and Get Pregnant Without Losing Your Mind*, witnessed the same problem in an ever more unfortunate circumstance:

"A friend undergoing testicular cancer treatment told me the hospital tried to set up a male support group, but no one showed up," she told me. "I think men are more action-oriented, generally speaking, and would like to solve the problem rather than process their feelings around it.

"Also, most men take their fertility for granted—so if there's a problem it's a shock to the system. (I think women are more prepared for the shock, because they've been warned about their biological clock.) It also ties into their concept—our concept—of masculinity, so it's more than just a medical problem . . . and how do you talk about *that*?"

———————

So if men won't talk to each other, is there another way for them to communicate, perhaps more anonymously?

The answer, thankfully, is yes.

Social media, as public as it is, has been a haven for men like British fertility patient Gareth Down. Down's infertility is classified as male factor, so he and his wife ended up using donor sperm. During the journey, Down looked into online groups, but ultimately didn't find a fit. So he created his own. Known as Men's Fertility Support, IVF/IUI/ICSI on Facebook, it bills itself as a "secure place for men only to talk."

"I started the group at the end of the process," Down says. "My wife had support throughout with groups; I dipped in and out of them but they were overwhelmingly full of posts from women, and I didn't feel my concerns were relevant to their posts to contribute. I was struggling with accepting the final round—it was cycle 9 and would be our last—out of money and fight, I was in a bad place."

Down, whose Facebook profile photo proudly shows him with his son, was at first ambivalent about starting up the group and becoming a spokesperson for it. "Initially the group was slow to take off, but after a few media campaigns with a fertility charity in the UK, it gained momentum," he said. "I am surprised it's the size it is now, but pleased it can help so many."

That size is indeed impressive. By mid-March 2020, the group stood at approximately 1,700 members, with hot topics ranging beyond fertility—Covid-19 concerns, relationship questions, and even masculinity itself.

Taking a spin through the posts amid a Messenger-based interview, I could instantly see just how effective the group was. From one lad (to borrow from UK vernacular) showing off his surroundings in the lab room to another updating statistics back from his embryologist to another summarizing the journey that led to success for him and his wife, the posts range from sentimental to satirical—yet the effect is surprisingly moving.

Other men-only groups have been launched by Fertility Matters Canada, where one in six couples struggle with infertility, and by RESOLVE in the US. Still, these efforts are a tiny fraction of the overall infertility support landscape. Witness, for example, *Matt and Doree's Eggcellent Adventure*. Hosting a popular podcast in the infertility community, the husband-and-wife duo spawned two Facebook support groups—one for the overall fertility community, which sat at roughly 5,800 members in March 2020, and a sister group for those who've had success and are now parents, which was 1,900 members strong at the same time. In both cases, unfortunately, the vast majority of posts and responses I saw were from female members. Does this mean that men aren't looking? Not necessarily—couples may be looking together, or male members may be quietly lurking; but either way, the number of men who are active on the platform is minimal.

There is an important dynamic to bear in mind when you compare a group like Matt and Doree's to Gareth Down's group. Some patients—presumably women as well as men—find it awkward to participate in non-gender-specific groups.

Chris Moorex has seen this firsthand. As a fertility patient alongside his wife, Moorex looked to Facebook for support but had difficulty finding a tribe there—in fact, he reports that he found hostility instead. Eventually, Moorex made his way to Down's male-only group, and knew he had a winner. "The online men's group has been amazing. I did join a few standard IVF groups to start, but to be honest, those groups are not a good place for men," Moorex explains over Facebook Messenger. "It's great [that] all the women can support each other, but often, even if not meant, most times there is quite a scathing reaction to guys: men not responding the way their partners think they should behave/think/act.

"The men's group gives a chance to ask questions, be heard—often questions you would never get the chance to ask anywhere else."

The online men's group format has been wildly successful in other online discussion forums, while accompanying resource guides have popped up across the Web. Yet even with the anonymity that the Internet can offer, men may still have trouble participating in discussions. Accordingly, other resources such as blogs and advice articles from professionals become that much more important.

Another medium that has helped many men get through their troubles is podcasts. Among those is the appropriately named *Male Infertility Podcast*. Host Nick Denton, as of mid-August 2020, had seventeen episodes recorded, interviewing guys from a variety of spaces, including support group leaders and fertility coaches. Occasionally Denton even dispenses his own advice.

Starting the podcast was a no-brainer for the non-obstructive azoospermia patient, whose family has expanded thanks to a sperm donor. "I do voiceover and also audiobook narrations, so I had the gear," Denton said. "I thought, how can I help the guys who are going through what I've been through, and am still going through? A podcast was the easiest way, plus I couldn't find a male-perspective podcast about infertility, so I made the *Male Infertility Podcast*, aka the *MIP*."

Conceiving the idea was one thing, but actually hitting the record button for the debut episode was another story. "I was nervous, [but] I was also eager to do my bit," he said. "I'd spoken to the wife about it a few weeks previously, and worked on what I want to say and do. I hadn't spoken to anyone in the media or online at all. Only family, friends and work colleagues."

Having resources like these is unquestionably important, so that men can hear (and tell) stories that inspire and encourage them. Particularly when few men in popular culture have spoken out about infertility— though this may finally be changing.

CHAPTER 26

I-U-AYE

One of the most difficult choices that a couple makes, once they are told they have to go the route of assisted reproductive technology—ART for short—is whether to jump straight into in vitro fertilization or explore other methods first. While many couples fear losing precious time, and likely having to ultimately undergo IVF anyway, there are several less invasive (and less expensive!) procedures that are certainly worth a look, depending on what factors might be causing your infertility.

Because ours was classified as unexplained, we were encouraged to explore everything, so before we broke the bank with full-blown IVF, we checked out a cheaper alternative, IUI.

IUI, or intrauterine insemination, is a pretty simple procedure where the sperm are injected into the female inside the uterus, close to the fallopian tubes. In essence, this eliminates the very not-male step of "asking for directions," and gives the little swimmers a light-rail ride right to where they need to go.

Still, once the sperm reach the fallopian tubes, they need to find the egg, wine and dine it, etc. What differentiates IUI from the classic turkey-baster method is that rather than injecting raw semen, the doctor retrieves sperm from the sample the male provides. Here's how the American Pregnancy Association describes it:

> *A semen sample will be washed by the lab to separate the semen from the seminal fluid. A catheter will then be used to insert the sperm directly into the uterus. This process maximizes the number of sperm cells that are placed in the uterus, thus increasing the possibility of conception.*[1]

So if you've ever heard a complaint that semen is dirty, you can now feel justified in the knowledge that, at least from a reproduction standpoint, it is.

Now, the good news about IUI:

1. It's minimally invasive.
2. It's affordable (comparatively speaking, of course).
3. It's efficient.

All told, an IUI procedure can take less than an hour, assuming the male can produce healthy semen in short order. The trick, though, is that said sperm must be produced on-site at the fertility lab you have selected; and I cannot stress this facet enough: when you are headed to, ahem, the production floor, make sure all equipment is in proper working order.

Allow me to elaborate.

As I described earlier, going through the rigors of semen production at the doctor's office is not an easy task. You're feeling like you're at the center of the universe, with a bright spotlight shone on you to make sure your swimmers are ready to go. As with other sperm donation situations, you must abstain from orgasm for a couple of days prior, and be of pretty sound health (a cold isn't the end of the world, but the flu can cause delay). Your female partner may be given hormone accelerators to ensure she is at her most fertile on the day of the procedure, and if you know anything about how those supplements can mess with a woman's moods, you'd better damn well be ready.

And so should the room.

See, the spot where I went to do the deed was not as prepared as I had hoped. Forget that the chair was fabric, forget that the magazines were from the 2000s (let alone that there were magazines, period, when Internet porn had been around for well over a decade). The real issue was the lighting.

Just as I got, ahem, into the groove, the lights began to flicker. At that point, the logical part of my brain should've said, "Hold up, something's not right here," but when you've held off for a few days, any logic is silenced, if not bound and gagged. I was too far to go back or to break. Interrupting the flow could have been a painful stoppage in play.

Sure as all heck, at that worst possible moment, the lights went out. Aiming became a literal shot in the dark. I did as best I could to fill the cup as much as I could, but . . . only a certain amount made it to the destination. Embarrassed (and likely swearing), I fumbled with the lights and finally got them working again, or at least long enough to clean up, pass my sample through the two-way cabinet, explain to the lovely nurse what had happened (and demonstrate how their light switch from the 1970s was failing), and return to my wife.

Explaining the situation was probably the hardest thing I have ever had to do. We shared a laugh, but it was nervous laughter. If I hadn't produced enough to get through the appointment, it would not only be the ultimate in "you had one job" humiliation, it would also mean another month of drugs and prep, and another draining trip to the clinic. I couldn't bear the thought.

Fortunately, by some miracle, enough had made it into the specimen cup that we were able to proceed. I owe this fully and completely to my abstaining from any sort of ejaculation not only for the recommended two days prior but an entire week. And when I say gone without, I don't just mean that orgasms were off the table. I'm talking full-out straight edge for the period. I have never been a smoker, I don't do drugs, and I abstained from beer, wine, the exercise bike, and the sauna to ensure I was as healthy as a horse on the big day. Let's face it—if somehow I botched this one (act of God/Electro aside), I would never live it down. I wasn't taking a single chance.

Unfortunately, and perhaps to the shock of no one, it didn't work.

IUI, folks, is relatively cheap, as I stated earlier. Ultimately, you're looking at the cost for drugs, five minutes of room rental for the guy, and a fairly straightforward injection of cleansed sperm. Your bill will likely be in the low four figures, depending on the drug protocol. The price, however, correlates with what is overall a pretty low success rate. VeryWellFamily produced a chart of success, which was divided by the age of the female (note: their statistics did not factor the quality or quantity of sperm).[2] The pregnancy rate was less than one in five for women between the ages of twenty and thirty, and less than 15 percent made it to term. The rate drops further for older women; after forty, it's 5.4 percent for pregnancy and 3 percent for delivery.

Nevertheless, because it is so inexpensive (again, by comparison), many couples will try it multiple times. We weren't willing to do that. At most, we were up for two sessions before moving on.

It's important to understand that IUI won't be recommended for every couple. Some people I spoke to told me that IUI was ruled out from the start, usually because the fallopian tubes were blocked or there wasn't a strong enough count of quality sperm available to make the procedure viable. Others stared blankly at me, never having even heard of the procedure.

There are other factors that come into play, such as precise timing, that can result in a failed IUI procedure, but I'll leave it to Dr. Aimee Eyvazzadeh to explain, courtesy of Medium.com:

"During IUI, roughly 50 million sperm cells are directed towards the egg. One would think that at just 3cm away (from the egg) it'd be quite simple for at least one sperm to fertilize an egg," Dr. Eyvazzadeh says in her article, "Why Isn't Your IUI Working?" "While I am the ultimate turkey baster, I am not a medical deity. The fact remains that human biology has its limitations."[3]

So if and when IUI doesn't work, you needn't walk away feeling ashamed. It is far from a miracle procedure. Any doctor will admit that.

But now comes the moment of truth, one so many couples have faced before you: the start of IVF.

CHAPTER 27

The Complete Idiot's Guide to IVF

The three letters most associated with infertility are I-V-F. Formally known as in vitro fertilization, IVF is what we kids of the '80s called the test-tube baby method. The process consists of quite literally forming an embryo outside of a woman's body, and then implanting it into her uterus for carriage and development.

The first step is to retrieve a woman's eggs. This requires taking preparatory hormone injections for about two weeks prior, but the procedure itself is brief and mostly painless. Generally, your doctor will try to extract as many eggs as possible for fertilization. The embryos will then mature for up to five days and be tested for viability (depending on the clinic, you will get a quality score on a scale of 10 or 20). The viable eggs will then be inserted into the womb. There are still debates as to whether it's best to implant one embryo or several, and some jurisdictions have strict rules for the sake of avoiding multiple births. So, first things first— know that if you are going to a clinic that will implant more than one embryo, there is the chance you will end up with twins (or more).

IVF is still a relatively young medical process; the first successful procedure was completed in 1978. Since then, as success rates improve, it has quickly gained a reputation as an infertility panacea. But the truth is much more complicated.

For one thing, IVF doesn't guarantee pregnancy and successful delivery. Age (of both male and female), health, and other factors come into play, along with the ability of the female to carry to full term. In fact, many couples will go through numerous rounds of IVF just for one successful pregnancy. Different clinics report different success rates, but perhaps even more important, they recommend different drug protocols.

So, let's talk drugs!

Unsurprisingly, the burden of hormone injections falls squarely on the female partner. This is where, with all due respect to my brothers, we as males should shut up, grin, and help our partners as much as possible. We're not the ones getting needles every night; we're not the ones being loaded with medication several times a day. Grin, bear it, and once you've produced your seed, have a beer, by all means.

Next is the almighty dollar factor, and when you're talking IVF, you're talking plenty of those. An IVF procedure, from start to finish, can easily range between $10,000 and $15,000 in North America, and most insurance won't cover a single aspect of it. To be honest, this has always boiled my blood, particularly in Canada, where most procedures are covered in part if not in full by our national healthcare system. The rationale for the exemption is that it's not "necessary" to have a kid. Sure, that may be the case, but it's also not "necessary" to have knee surgery—you *elect* to have it done so you can walk again at full capacity. You *could* walk with an aid, the same way that a hopeful parent *could* wait to become an uncle or an aunt, but do you think you should have to use a cane at forty (or sixty, for that matter?). I rest my case.

There is one part of the process, however, that *may* be covered, and that's the aforementioned drug protocol. This was something I learned when my wife and I were prepping for IVF. At the time, I was working for a marketing agency, and, before we went in for our procedure, I put in a call to our group benefits rep to see if any of the protocol would be covered. Turns out, the language in our plan worked to my benefit. You see, if your drug plan does not explicitly say that a drug you or your partner is prescribed is meant for the purpose of infertility treatments, you're free to submit it. The savings? A few thousand bucks. Nothing to sneeze at!

Given the costliness, especially relative to the success rates, how common is IVF? In a 2018 report, Penn Medicine found that in 2012, just under 62,000 babies were born in the US as a result of IVF.[1] So in other words, you could fill a football stadium with screaming, crying IVF babies every year. (And yes, chances are they would be better behaved than the Raider Nation. Just saying.)

Now, there's one more IVF myth I should debunk here. During a Google search on "IVF and Men," under the People Also Ask tab, one of the listed questions was, "Can you guarantee a boy with IVF?" Obviously, the answer is no, but back in 2010, the BBC reported on an Australian study that found the odds of having a boy increased from 51/100 to 56/100 when IVF was used. This, however, was not the case if ICSI was involved. There, you were more likely to have a girl.

What's ICSI, you ask? Glad you did! We're all about the handy acronyms here.

ICSI, or intracytoplasmic sperm injection, injects a single sperm into an egg, past the outer layer, which cannot always be penetrated. This is in contrast to a standard IVF process, whereby, according to the American Society for Reproductive Medicine, "50,000 or more swimming sperm are placed next to the egg in a laboratory dish. Fertilization occurs when one of the sperm enters into the cytoplasm of the egg."[2]

This isn't quite the "tuck" or "no tuck" dilemma George Costanza faced—it's a little less trivial. The ASRM states that ICSI greatly increases your chances of fertilization—to as much as 50 to 80 percent. You can't help but like those odds! But ICSI does carry a higher rate of major birth defects than natural conception (as does IVF in general), and it costs more. Some folks probably think of it as buying a few extra numbers to increase your odds at getting the house you want—especially since there's always a good chance you'll need more than one round of standard IVF.

Now, more about those drugs. The truth is, they can make all the difference in the world. Depending on what medical conditions you or your partner have, the protocol can be quite simple or exceedingly complicated. The key is to find a doctor you have full faith and confidence in.

It was for this reason that our fertility journey led out of Winnipeg.

After our round of IUI failed, our doctor didn't try to steer us in any particular direction, instead saying it was up to us what we did next.

Great. Thanks.

We could have done IVF in Winnipeg, but since our doctor wasn't inspiring much confidence, we decided to open things up. Our research suggested there were a few options available, both in Canada and the US. Ultimately, we chose Victoria, British Columbia, where we found doctors inclined toward deeper, more experimental drug protocols that looked beyond Clomid and letrozole to underlying conditions that may be affecting your ability to conceive, such as autoimmune conditions.

Was I nervous when we had our first consult over Skype? You bet. My wife was gung-ho, but I was a little wary. Going to Victoria meant being away for nearly a month, and there was no way of knowing whether what they were proposing would work.

In the end, though, I didn't see a lot of alternatives. We could have done another round of IUI, but it would be a total crapshoot, and likely waste a few thousand dollars (since the rate of success is much lower than for IVF and we would still have to travel after losing faith in our local fertility clinic). If we were going to stay on this road, I wanted it to lead somewhere.

So we packed up the Toyota and headed west.

CHAPTER 28

The Road You Travel for Fertility

Depending on where you live, there may be a fertility treatment center around every corner, or fewer than a handful.

Because fertility is, for the most part, not publicly funded (or even covered by most private insurance), finding clinics can be hard. Even in Canada, ART is not really funded. Some provinces offer some coverage, but generally not beyond a single round. More to the point, you can't go into a hospital and have IVF done.

If you're in a metropolis like Toronto, you don't have much of an issue, but in Winnipeg, at least as of 2020, there was still only one facility. Poetically, it's about a two-minute drive from the radio station where "Greg" made his public debut.

The facility was our first step on our fertility journey, but it wasn't our last. After trying a few different processes, including drugs and IUI (remember my "lights out" moment?), nothing had worked. And we weren't getting much guidance on what to do next. Joy.

To put this in perspective, imagine going into swimming lessons for the first time. You head into the pool excited and ready to earn that yellow badge, or whatever the system is these days. What you find is a horrible teacher who pushes your head underwater when you complain about opening your eyes beneath the surface and how much the chlorine is burning (in case you can't tell, this happened to me when I was all of five years old). As you exit the water, traumatized, your parents will likely explore other options to get their child trained. As a child, you'd count on their expertise and knowledge to lead you so you don't end up at the bottom of a lake.

Feel like you're drowning just from the stress? That's what we felt like, too. Another round of IUI? IVF—with or without ICSI? More drugs? It was like we were standing in line at McDonald's instead of a medical facility. Is it bad enough that we should consider surrogacy? Just keep trying naturally until our collective spirit is completely broken?

At this point, we knew we were going to need to travel, like so many other couples before us. It happens a lot more than you probably think. Whether you have no clinic within your immediate region or just aren't getting the service you expected, there are plenty of reasons to look around. Couples that we met during our journey went as far as the Czech Republic for their procedure. (For those wondering, Zlin is apparently a wonderful haven for egg donors.)

When we made the decision to look elsewhere, we had a few options. Being close to the US border, Fargo, North Dakota, was a strong possibility, and we had heard great things about their facilities; but ultimately we chose to stay in Canada. After reviewing Calgary, Montreal, and Toronto, we had our first consultation with the Victoria Fertility Clinic out in British Columbia. After one meeting with our would-be doctor, we were hooked; as it turned out, we weren't the only Winnipeggers who had chosen this clinic. In fact, one of our fellow support group couples arrived mere days before we left.

Within most families, there are varying comfort levels with travel. My wife was a big-time road-tripper from birth. Her family moved to the US for a year when her father took a job in Tulsa, and her family occasionally visited her grandparents in Florida, making the cross-continent trek by car. My family, on the other hand, had only driven as far as Chicago, once, preferring to stick to North Dakota and Minnesota. (Note for audio copy: this is when TLC's "Waterfalls" should be playing.)

There was no option for us to go by plane or train, since we were going to be housed in Victoria for a full month (less a couple of days when I needed to fly back and forth for work). That meant packing up much of our house and lives and heading for an Airbnb.

I've never been much of a travel writer, but I can tell you this—driving *to* Victoria, ferry included, in the middle of October is a hell of a lot simpler than driving *from* Victoria in November. But more on this in a moment.

It was never going to be an easy ride, particularly with an overanxious dog. My wife had just started her stimulation injections, and would have to do several en route to our destination. So nerves were running high, especially when we almost missed the ferry from Canada's mainlaind to Vancouver Island. Along the way we had a few unique experiences, including when we arrived in Medicine Hat, Alberta, for our first night, only to learn that our booking platform didn't get the message properly to the hotel that we needed a room that was pet friendly. We could've argued, but after seeing a drug deal go down behind the building, we got back on the road.

Despite all that, the drive was beautiful. We stopped at a couple of places along the way to enjoy the sights of western Canada. For a prairie boy, driving directly through mountain ranges was a thrill. I did the likely illegal but very worth-it move of setting my phone up in a holster so I could snap pictures as I drove up and down the winding highways that make up the Coquihalla. Incidentally, if you have never driven on this pathway, don't—it's windy, narrow, and has terrible cell phone reception (at least it did in 2014).

By the time we reached our temporary basement home, I was ready to relax. Victoria, aside from the rainstorms—which are soak-you-to-the-bone cold and fierce—is a beautiful part of Canada, with beaches, urban farms, unique boutiques, and absolutely the friendliest people on the planet. I'm sorry, Winnipeg, but when a Victoria traffic cop leaves a note on your window that you didn't pay for parking properly with a Ferrero Rocher attached, you just can't compete.

Victoria also had all the amenities I could ever want. Mid-production on a book (which I won't name since it was with another publisher, but you can check out my Amazon author page to learn more), I sat in a café that was a three-minute walk from the clinic and wrote for hours on end. The only thing I really missed was my Xbox, but I couldn't complain. Every day after my work was done, we would take our dog to the lake for a walk and plan dinner.

The serenity of Victoria certainly helped with our preparations, but so did simply escaping the hustle and bustle of our everyday lives. It was almost like we could pretend to be different people for three weeks and approach our first appointment as a fresh start.

During the trip, I had all of one beer, and never took out the bike I our Airbnb hosts had left for us. No way was I taking any chances. I could celebrate endlessly later, but considering my direct contribution to the IVF procedure would last all of five minutes, I was going to have it but-toned up.

And honestly, I didn't need anything. I didn't crave alcohol like I did when I was out with my buddies at home, or grilling in our backyard. Again, it's amazing how much a change of scenery can transform your mindset.

Anyway, my point is, if you have any sort of inkling that the clinic near you is not the right fit, don't use it. The cliché about having the best chance at baby success when you're calm has a certain truth to it, but in the case of being able to choose where you go through IVF or other ARTs, even if you're just doing a three-hour drive across provincial or state lines, do it. Being outside your routine and making a holiday out of your journey is one of the best things you could ever do. Some couples have gone as far as traveling from Canada to Europe for treatments and made a full travelogue out of their infertility journey.

For many couples, the cause behind the travel is financial. Witness the findings by CNBC in 2019. Writer Megan Leonhardt (who for some reason identified in her title that *Women*, not *Couples* or *Women and Men*, are traveling for IVF treatments) reported that thousands of couples travel across the US for the most affordable IVF treatment.[1] Leonhardt shared the story of Anna and her husband, a Los Angeles couple, who crossed the country to Albany, New York, for a $20,000 procedure. They were able to reduce some of their costs by getting creative. "To keep her expenses as low as possible, Anna ordered the priciest medications from Israel and purchased others through discounts she found using GoodRx," Leonhardt reported. "Plus she paid for her IVF using a newly acquired credit card to snag a promotional points offer. Those points paid for the flights to and from New York, as well as accommodations and a rental car."

Another way to ease the financial burden, incidentally, is to look at benefits available to you. There can be some provisions in tax law that you can speak with an accountant about, or insurance providers, such as those that provide the health plan for your employer, that may be able to find loopholes for you.

Others will simply take the opportunity to make a full experience out of the IVF travel. You've heard of some couples taking "babymoons" just before the arrival of a child? Well, this is one step earlier, sometimes called an IVF vacation or, as CTV News wittily called it, the "procreation vacation." The Canadian news network spoke with the Barbados Fertility Centre, which reported that 14 percent of their patients are Canadian.[2] The successful birth rate at this clinic? According to the clinic's medical director, Dr. Juliet Skinner, it's pretty damn high. "Under [the age of] 35, we have a 67 per cent success rate, and a 57 per cent for over 35. With egg donors, we have a 75 per cent success rate."

Ahem, two piña coladas, please, but make them virgin . . .

The unfortunate side effect of all this travel, whether you call it cross-border fertility or fertility vacations, is the loss both in business and reputation to your local fertility economy. When we traveled to Victoria, we weren't the only Winnipeg couple that did so. Not only, historically, had the BC capital received many patients from our prairie province, but as we were preparing to leave the island, another couple from our fertility group was arriving. Others went to Calgary, Toronto, and even the Czech Republic for procedures, because their needs weren't being met locally or they felt that getting away would be a huge benefit to them.

"[Getting away] is a big draw for patients," says Dr. Eleanor Stevenson. "You can say, 'I want to go to Thailand, we can get a trip, sit on the beach, get stimulated, have IVF, come home cheaper, pregnant and had a lovely vacation, with a little bit of sunburn.' I can totally see the benefit of that. I would suggest we need to, as a healthcare system, do a better job of providing situations where the same benefit that comes—that addition of counterbalancing a stressful time with my mental health, where you don't feel like you need that vacation."

Not everything we did in Victoria was fun and games, of course. We were there for a reason, after all. There were certainly anxious moments, not least as I abstained as long as I could from any sexual activity, particularly on the days leading up to my five minutes of fame. If there was one thing I most definitely was not going to do, it was risk everything on the trip for a few minutes of enjoyment. Injecting my wife with needles every night, I had to learn on the fly how to just stick it in and be quick about it.

But on the big day, thankfully, the protocol was simple. While my wife was having her eggs extracted, I was going to take care of my end of the bargain. Thankfully, this setup was much better—a leather chair, a TV with an endless stream of entertainment, Wi-Fi, and most important, working lights! And this time, things went swimmingly.

Once I was done, I joined my wife in the extraction room. The egg count was, happily, very high. I will not downplay the importance of this, because many women who either have trouble with production or have other factors in their infertility produce a minimal amount of eligible eggs (six or fewer), making the whole process that much more fraught.

We then waited five days while the eggs were fertilized, frozen, and matured. As you can imagine, it was excruciating. I knew that just because we had successfully created the two parts of the equation, it didn't necessarily mean the embryos would be ready to go. The scale Victoria used for viability ranged from 1 to 20, and any embryo that scored less than a 15 would not be approved for implantation. Further, those deemed strong enough would have to go through rounds of genetic testing to avoid any potentially negative situations. (This is extremely important if you or your partner has a condition in your genetic history that can be life-altering, or not discovered until later in life.) This process can be controversial, as you are, to an extent, "playing God," but genetic testing has become common practice even for couples conceiving naturally, and certainly for us it was about knowledge and comfort, not, say, choosing the baby's gender (which you actually can do in some jurisdictions, by the way).

There are other facets to the overall equation and it can't be emphasized enough that just because you can make eggs, that doesn't mean implantation can just happen. There are so many working parts that come into play. Even a misstep in accelerated cycle can mean the difference between implantation and waiting a month.

After the five-day wait, we had nine embryos that were deemed eligible. Naturally, we weren't taking any chances, and chose to implant the strongest. And yes, I mean the single strongest, as our clinic's policy was to implant only one embryo (which would have been our preference in any case).

The night before implantation day, we did all the things a pregnant woman can't do: went for terrific sushi (and yes, it's *much* better on the coast!), had some wine, and enjoyed a quiet evening. The next day was going to be somewhat stressful, both because of implantation and the unfortunate timing that I had to be headed back to Winnipeg that night for work. If I didn't have to be in town for meetings, I would much rather have taken the time to stay the extra few days in Victoria, but it wasn't feasible.

And so, there we were all scrubbed up and ready for the implantation. Our regular doctor, unfortunately, wasn't with us, but his partner was terrific. Before the embryo was implanted, it flashed on a TV screen in the procedure room. Not many couples can say they have photos of their kids at minus-forty weeks, but there she was for us to see. It was heartwarming, and the attachment was immediate.

After a couple of hours' rest at the clinic, I had to head back to Winnipeg for work. I boarded the plane more anxious than I had ever been in my life. Despite all the promises and prospects, all the medication and preparation, could something happen while I was away? What if the doctors did something wrong?

This is the part that truly sucks about traveling for infertility. Unless you are able to completely put your life on hold, either there are parts that will come with you or you'll have to cut your trip short at some point. Though remote work is suddenly much more of a reality in our post-coronavirus world, back in 2014, I was expected on the ground at home. I still had clients who needed their meetings, and operations that could only be done in person.

And so, reluctantly, after the procedure was done and I sat with my resting wife as long as I could, I made the solo trip back to Winnipeg, where work, bills, and family waited for me. I can remember most of the flights I've taken in my life—the time a couple offered up their window seat to me so they could sit side by side (and later escape to the bathroom together); the ultra-chatty woman who spilled wine on my copy of the *Hockey News* and paid for my drink to apologize; my tray table pushed into my stomach as a sleeping passenger leaned back in his seat amid a twelve-hour, understaffed flight between Amsterdam and Toronto. But this one I honestly cannot recall at all. Nerves were too high, and I'm pretty sure I passed out midway through.

Keeping in close touch for the next few days was tough. On top of my meetings, snow was on its way, so I had to prep our outdoor setup and make sure we had some food in the fridge. My wife, meanwhile, had our dog with her for company. God bless the little weiner, he's always been the best cuddle buddy you could ever ask for. He helped us at many points along the journey, but never more crucially than those few days.

After roughly a week in Winnipeg, I flew back to Victoria to repack our car for the drive home. We decided to take the long way home, stopping first in Salmon Lake, BC, for a night before moving on to Calgary, where my wife would get a blood test. The weather, unfortunately, had taken a turn for the worse, as fall gave way to winter. Virtually as soon as we hit the BC–Alberta border, a blizzard engulfed us. We saw one semi in the ditch along the highway, and at least one tree had cracked and collapsed. No, this was certainly not Chinook weather. If you've ever wondered what white-knuckle driving would feel like, imagine being hit suddenly by a few good inches of snow, not letting go of the steering wheel as you plow through with an overanxious dog barking at the feet of your pregnant wife. Let's just say that I was never happier to see boring, flat prairie land than I was when we hit Regina roughly thirty-six hours later.

Wait, did I say pregnant?? Yep, I did.

About forty-five minutes after we docked in Vancouver, we got the call we'd been desperate for. The IVF procedure was a success, and my wife (not we) was on her way to having a baby.

CHAPTER 29

The Second Miscarriage and Secondary Infertility

We're winding down a Disney cruise in the fall of 2019 as I write this chapter.

As has happened all week, my daughter fell asleep at dinner. Determined parents that we are, however, we're keeping her out of bed so that we can see a show before we make port in the morning.

My wife has been looking forward to this cruise for ages. Disney has the uncanny ability to attract everyone from singles to friends to newlyweds to seniors, but it's parents of young children, naturally, who flock in the greatest numbers. No other franchise has ever come close to the enduring appeal. Put mouse ears in just about any other context (especially a kitchen floor) and you do not get a favorable reaction. Contenders to the animated thrown and imitators have come and gone, but none compare to the power of the celebrated mouse and co. Bugs Bunny and the Looney Tunes crew don't have the cachet they once did. Even the Mighty and Danger versions of the animated rodents have not survived. Yet Mickey, Minnie, and their cast of friends . . . they aren't parents themselves, mind you (save for Goofy and the horridly annoying *Goof Troop* cast), yet they are, for the most part, uncles or aunts.

But the trip is only partially celebratory. It's also meant to be cleansing, a time to refresh, as we move on from the last attempt to build our family.

Earlier in the year my wife and I returned to Victoria for a second round of IVF. For various reasons, we had waited a while before pursuing a second child, even as our friends mostly became families of four. Admittedly, I was way more hesitant than the first time, and I had sort of resigned myself to being the parent of a single child. But there was also the part of me that did want a second kid, in part because both my wife and I had grown up with siblings we loved.

The second round was, of course, less stressful than the first. We didn't have to drive on the Coquihalla or inject an insane amount of drugs beforehand—and, of course, there was zero performance anxiety. We still had several embryos frozen from the first round, and one would be used in this cycle. We were only going to be there for a few days, so rather than Airbnb it like we had previously, we stayed at a cozy seaside resort with a few decent walking trails and a restaurant nearby. Implantation day went smoothly, and we rested from then on while our daughter stayed with her grandparents.

A couple of weeks later, we found out the procedure was successful, but just as before, we were cautious. A few friends knew, but we were mostly quiet about it, keeping our fingers crossed.

Then, while at a friend's wedding in another city, we had to make an emergency run to a rural hospital as my wife miscarried.

Earlier, I talked about how I was frozen during the first miscarriage. This was different. I was a lot more emotional; I sobbed openly. I had prepared for the worst, in a sense, but I felt more defeated than ever.

Going through loss the second time around reminded me of how difficult life with infertility is. There's the feeling of accomplishment, no matter how many cycles you've been through, when it appears you may be successful again. Some couples I've known naturally conceived after initially having to use ART or adopted. The old wives' tale is that this is because you are more relaxed. (I don't buy that theory, personally.)

Still, multiple rounds of IVF or other procedures are the reality for many families, and not just those who've had trouble all along; secondary infertility is common for couples who conceived naturally the first time as well.

Witness, for example, Margaret Renkl. Writing for *Parents* magazine, Renkl disclosed that her first child came virtually by accident. She and her beau were almost cocky in their belief that a second child, this time intended, would come quickly. It didn't.

"After all, if I could conceive without meaning to, how hard could it be to get pregnant on purpose? We'd just grin at each other one afternoon during the baby's nap, and a few weeks later a little blue line would magically appear in the window of a pregnancy test," she wrote. "Two years and two miscarriages later, we had learned a sad lesson in human biology: Fertility is not always within our control."[1]

Secondary infertility can happen for any number of reasons. According to the Mayo Clinic,[2] they include:

- Impaired sperm production, function, or delivery in men
- Fallopian tube damage, ovulation disorders, endometriosis, and uterine conditions in women
- Complications related to prior pregnancy or surgery
- Changes in risk factors for you or your partner, such as age, weight, and use of certain medications

Secondary infertility can damage a relationship just as much as primary; in fact, the surprise factor can be particularly devastating. However, with infertility that comes after success the first time around, there is a compounded feeling, in large part because past success should, theoretically, mean that another conception should be likely. As a result, as discussed by UW Health on its Generations fertility care website in 2019, relationships can become strained, just as they do for primary infertility cases.[3]

"The stress of secondary infertility on an individual's life and relationships can be significant. It can be hard to find support from family and friends, especially when a woman or couple already has/have children. Sentiments such as, 'you should be grateful for what you have,' or, 'just keep trying,' almost never serve as useful advice or support," the site states. "Couples and single parents can even experience resentment from other couples with infertility who are unable to have even one child."

Equally important, your child may have strong feelings around secondary infertility. Explaining to our daughter, who was excited to have a brother or sister, that we weren't going to have one (yet, at least) was difficult. She mourned just as much as, if not more than, we did. Even months after the miscarriage, she would talk about it from time to time, surfacing our own feelings of grief, not to mention guilt.

We have to remember that children are more intuitive than we give them credit for, and their emotions are just as powerful as ours are. We should make sure they know that secondary infertility is not a result of anything they did or didn't do.

"Because children can pick up on their parents' stress, it is also important to pay attention to how their kids may be feeling," UW Health continues. "Children might not understand why their parents are feeling a certain way, and attribute it to something they've done."

Unsurprisingly, solving secondary infertility can be tricky, especially since you're already juggling the responsibility of one child. "Have you been on top of the preconception game, or are you just too busy for baby-planning activities like charting and timing baby-making sex (or any sex for that matter)? Given that you have a little one underfoot, it's understandable if you're more exhausted than ever," wrote Sharon Mazel on whattoexpect.com, on the subject of secondary infertility.[4] "It's not easy for wannabe second-time parents to devote as much time and energy to TTC as they likely did on the first go-around, but it would be helpful to take a step back (and a hard look) at what's going on."

So what *can* we do? Mazel advises that your kid(s) can actually be a huge help. "In the midst of your infertility problems, you may feel especially upset about shifting your focus from the child you already have to the child you're longing to have in the future. You may even feel guilty about your inability to give your little one a sibling or about the sadness you are sure is spilling over into her life," she wrote. "The best thing you can do for your child in this situation is to keep life as normal as possible, and ideally, find some quality time to be together. Whether it's a chat about her day before you tuck her into bed or an afternoon romp in the park, those rituals will go a long way toward keeping your tot's world stable and happy—even if you sometimes feel your world is spinning out of control."

Admittedly, we had a much different experience the second time around because we had a wider circle of people going through the same struggle. Those who were on the primary infertility journey with us had, for the most part, stopped at that first child; but now, as we approached forty, there was a new set experiencing infertility for the first time. Because we had already been so public, we found a new tribe to talk with and share our feelings with openly. Even those friends who had gone on to have more children felt more aligned with us because they had witnessed our struggle so directly.

Still, it did hurt when I saw others succeed. I was quietly conscious of which families were growing. No, I wasn't hoping for a boy—I didn't need to carry on the family name or crave father-son bonding moments. I would've been happy with a second daughter, even if it meant getting crowded out of the bathroom twice as often.

Ultimately, secondary infertility can be as painful as primary, and just like that first round, you have to decide as a couple how far you're willing to go. Luckily, there's more awareness than ever that families come in every shape and size. And if we're meant to be complete with our one little angel, I'll be more than satisfied.

CHAPTER 30

It Doesn't Go Away

Back in 2015, even after our pregnancy was confirmed, we held off on celebrating too much; after all, we knew by now that miscarriage can occur even months later. Once we were finally clear of that proverbial danger zone, we made the announcement we had waited so long for—and because it was 2015, we did it over Facebook.

Pregnancy was an adventure, as anyone who has gone through it will tell you. Just about every urban legend you hear is true, and if you're lucky, your community wants to celebrate you with showers and gifts.

When we made our announcement, people came out of the woodwork just as much as they had when we first started sharing our story. The Facebook algorithm is a tricky one—even for a digital marketing specialist—to decipher. You can be "friends" with people through the network yet never see a post from them. But suddenly I was hearing from those folks, sharing their joy for us.

It felt great, but in truth, even the milestone of pregnancy brought with it a sense of isolation. Leave aside, just for a moment, that sentiment people share of "we're so happy that it finally happened for you!"

I'll get back to that in a few moments. There were times in the pregnancy that both of us still felt, for lack of a better term, different.

As much as I wanted to celebrate, I worried that the "I" word would shadow us forever. Because the struggle to conceive had been so great, we couldn't shake that feeling of being extra cautious, on guard. It was as if we had summited a mountain but weren't able to climb back down to the safety of the flat land. Instead, there were still stigmas attached. At least, being not devotedly religious, we were spared most whispering about how our baby came to be—in fact, we held our daughter's naming ceremony at our synagogue, in the same room where we'd signed our marriage contract.

Some of this discomfort, of course, comes from the sentiment I described above—"finally." For me, it triggered the same feeling as my classmate's "you'd better catch up" two years earlier. You want to be just like any other pregnant couple, but even in your own eyes, you aren't.

And, of course, once you've successfully given birth to a child, it doesn't take long for people to ask when you're going to try for a second.

Let's hit pause for a moment here, because there is a semi-myth that should be addressed. I, like many others in the infertility community, have heard the stories of "well, they adopted and then had the second one naturally!" For those couples, and I do know a few, I say congratulations; but just like the couple who get pregnant while awaiting their spot for IVF, it's more the exception than the rule.

The reality is that whether you adopt, go through ART, or have your first child through some other means, your body (and mind) don't suddenly reset. Mario can start a new level as fresh as a daisy; infertile couples don't.

But that was a subject to address later. For now, we sat in a parenting class put on by one of the local baby boutiques. It's a brilliant marketing concept, really: bring X number of soon-to-be parents into a gathering room in your store so they can check out your designer wares, from bibs to booties.

Even weeks from giving birth, I felt isolated from so many other parents. A few friends who knew our story were with us, but so, too, were acquaintances who didn't. I know it sounds crazy, but it felt as isolating there as it did in high school being an average student in a class of overachievers. Even if it was just my psyche playing games with me (as was likely the case), I felt so alone, because of how our path was different. I loved my daughter-to-be as much as the next dad, but I felt myself clutch up in the moment, overwhelmed with anxiety.

Turns out, I probably wasn't the only one. In a 2019 article for the *New York Times* called "The Lasting Trauma of Infertility," Regina Townsend talked about her own journey, which included a failed adoption and ultimately IVF. When she wrote the article, then six months a mother, she still felt like she was suffering the ill effects of the ordeal, even as she held her new son. "I should have felt invincible, but instead, I was numb. I felt as if the other shoe would drop at any moment. I had to pay for the victory that was my son, didn't I? That was the routine of the roller coaster infertility had been for us. No success without swift defeat," she wrote. "Fire can leave serious damage behind. Because it can be hard to fully grasp what infertility involves unless you've dealt with it personally, many people believe that it's all about the end game, a baby—that if you could just get to that prize, the pain of infertility would fade away. But infertility is bigger than babies. I say this often, because I want people to get it. It truly is. It can affect our physical and mental health in insidious—and sometimes enduring—ways.

"Indeed, going through infertility, even coming out successful on the other side, had ever-lasting effects that I can best describe as PTSD. You can't just go back to 'normalcy' of life before infertility entered your life, the same way that most soldiers cannot go back to the every day once they return from battle. The experience changes the way you view yourself, the people you know and the world around you."[1]

I couldn't agree more. I realized that, no matter how much my wife and I had in common with every other team of first-time parents in the room, it would help if there were a support group for expecting or new parents who had struggled with infertility. But there wasn't. Our local support chapter had a virtual parents group, where folks could message each other, but nothing with regular meetings and engagement.

The community, however, stayed with us in one important way. Shortly after we announced our successful pregnancy, three other couples we were friends with as part of our support group announced they were pregnant as well. All in all, by Labor Day (pardon the pun), four IVF babies were going to be crying and pooping in Winnipeg.

So what did we do? Rather than hide away or ignore our feelings, we embraced them. Just a few months into her life, our daughter met the babies who, like her, were born in a realm beyond hope. In the basement of a community library, in late October, those four babies lay in their tiny Halloween costumes. I don't think any other tykes, perhaps short of the Dionne Quintuplets, have had as many photos taken at such a tender age in the space of three minutes. And it wasn't just moms, babies, and me— all the proud dads were in the room, sharing stories of the cute things our kids had already done while also prognosticating the success of our beloved Jets for the remainder of the hockey season.

Elsewhere in the room, older kids, also of IVF origin, played in their own ways. My wife had lugged in countless toys for everyone to play with and set up stations for coloring, blocks, and other activities. It was a moment of deep satisfaction that we repeated for several years, each time adding more successful families.

Our tribe had come together, and were standing happy that day. As a father, I was never prouder—or less alone.

Epilogue

It's Labor Day 2020, the unofficial end to the most bizarre summer in recorded history. Already, in Winnipeg, the weather has turned cool enough for mitts and a toque as you walk down the street.

Today, unlike my venture to the radio station all those years ago, I'm not alone. My wife and daughter are with me, as is a friend who just had her own IVF miracle baby, right smack in the middle of Covid's first wave.

It's a reflective time for me, the summer before the child I sometimes thought I would never have enters kindergarten. We're trying to savor the last few days before the reality of "school" amid the coronavirus pandemic hits us fully in the face.

That summer we spent three weeks in cottage country, and I did the things I had always longed to do with a kid of my own—toss a ball around, ride bikes with my daughter (and dog) in the chariot, go downtown for ice cream, throw rocks into the creek, bore her with tales of yesteryear, chase frogs, watch cartoons, play video games, roast marshmallows, and relax on the beach. There were also some activities I wasn't as excited about, like camping in the backyard, but hey, parenthood.

The true highlight for me was taking out the family canoe with my daughter and three of her cousins. Five of us in a heavier-than-believable watercraft. I've known all three cousins since they were born, as many as fifteen years ago, and all three of them have known my daughter since she arrived in 2015. It's these rare moments of pure tranquility that made me so envious for so many years.

Soon, the leaves will turn colors, fall, and be pulled into piles for my daughter to jump in for all of three days before we're encased in a couple of feet of snow for a few months. That's life in Canada.

This Labor Day has its own peace. Covid be damned, it's a day when most Winnipeggers will walk outside, smile, and say "hello" to each other, even though we're perfect strangers. We took plenty of those walks this summer, with neighbors commenting on my daughter's beautiful hair (of course, they've never had to tame her curls after a bath).

As we walk and talk, my innocent child, who is obsessed with weddings, princesses, and L.O.L. Surprise dolls, pipes up with one of her signature questions.

"How do babies get in the mommy's tummy?" she asks, full of wonder.

Kiddo, have I got an answer for you.

Acknowledgments

This was, by far, the most intense book I've ever written, and certainly the most personal (though that's an easy accomplishment, given that I was never a member of the Winnipeg Jets, was never a wrestler, and do not have my own baseball card . . . yet).

Working on such a personal project is consuming in so many ways, and would not have been possible without the patience, care, and support of my wife, Elana, and my daughter, Kaia. There were times I had to sequester myself to finish chapters or just play mindless video games to get my thoughts going through mental roadblocks. I thank you from the bottom of my heart and love you both immeasurably. Thank you to our dog, Mercer, too, who knew when I needed a cuddle as I faced some tough chapters, and to my family and friends, who let me drone on about the book-writing experience.

I also want to thank the good people at Tiller Press and Simon & Schuster, starting with Sam Ford, who was the first to see value in taking a chance on a man writing about infertility. It's a far cry from our usual conversations for certain. Thank you, next, to my editor, Emily Carleton, who was encouraging and an excellent guide through the process. I cannot recommend her enough as an editor for anyone lucky enough to work with her (LinkedIn nod coming).

Next, I want to thank the media, who have allowed me to share my story and speak about infertility over the years. I'm fortunate at this point to have done so many interviews that it would be an exceedingly long list of names, but most of you know who you are and know that my thanks are sincere. I do have to single out Dahlia Kurtz, though, as she was the one who gave me my voice in the first place and let me hide out as "Greg." I say this with sincerity—look up her audio archive—she is one of the most genuine people in media.

I'd like to thank my gracious interviewees for making this book possible: "Lolly," Amy Klein, Amy Weber, Annie Kuo, Chris Moorex, Dr. Eleanor Stevenson, Gareth Down, Greg Sdeo, Greg Sommer, Josh Huber, Karen Jeffries, Kate Brian, Dr. Kevin McEleney, Liberty Barnes, Mike Heller, Nick Denton, Spencer and Whiteney Blake, Tracey Sainsbury, and Vince Londini.

I know I'm not alone in this one, but thanks definitely have to go to Dr. Stephen Hudson in Victoria. It was because of Dr. Hudson and his staff that we have Kaia. Dr. Hudson is now enjoying retirement, and I know that there are so many patients who feel the same immense gratitude as my family.

I also want to extend thank-yous to the incredible team at TEDx Winnipeg. Many of you knew that my end goal was this book (and beyond). I share this with my coaches and fellow speakers.

Last but certainly not least, thank you to the infertility community for your support and willingness to either be interviewed or share thoughts with me.

Notes

Prologue

1. Julia Belluz, "Sperm Counts Are Falling. This Isn't the Reproductive Apocalypse—Yet," *Vox*, May 30, 2019, https://www.vox.com/science-and -health/2018/9/17/17841518/low-sperm-count-semen-male-fertility.

Chapter 2: Miscarriage of Justice

1. "Infertility and Miscarriage," NewLife Fertility Centre, https://newlifefer tility.com/get-started/infertility-and-miscarriage/.
2. "Multiple Miscarriage," RESOLVE: The National Infertility Association, https://resolve.org/infertility-101/medical-conditions/multiple-miscarriage/.
3. Raymond Baxter, "Men and Miscarriage," *Sammiches & Psych Meds* (blog), https://www.sammichespsychmeds.com/men-and-miscarriage/.
4. Adriel Booker, "Men & Miscarriage Series: Do Men and Women Grieve Differently after Pregnancy Loss?" AdrielBooker.com, July 7, 2018, http:// adrielbooker.com/miscarriage-men-women-grieve-differently/.

Chapter 3: Defining Infertility

1. Mohammad Reza Sadeghi, "Unexplained Infertility, the Controversial Matter in Management of Infertile Couples," *Journal of Reproduction & Infertility* 16, no. 1 (January–March 2015): 1–2, https://www.ncbi.nlm.nih.gov/pmc /articles/PMC4322174/.
2. "What Is Male Infertility?" Urology Care Foundation, https://www.urology health.org/urologic-conditions/male-infertility.

3. "Diagnosis: Infertility," National Health Service (UK), https://www.nhs.uk/conditions/infertility/diagnosis/.

4. "Endometriosis," US Department of Health & Human Services, Office on Women's Health, https://www.womenshealth.gov/a-z-topics/endometriosis.

Chapter 4: Starting a Journey

1. Sherrie Campbell, "6 Ways to Take the First Step of Your Journey to Success," *Entrepreneur*, January 21, 2016, https://www.entrepreneur.com/article/269794.

Chapter 5: Frozen in Time

1. Andrea Thompson, "Bad Memories Stick Better Than Good," Live Science, September 5, 2007, https://www.livescience.com/1827-bad-memories-stick-good.html.

Chapter 6: What Causes Male Infertility

1. Children's National Health System, "Experimental Fertility Preservation Provides Hope for Young Men," ScienceDaily, May 23, 2019, www.sciencedaily.com/releases/2019/05/190523184938.htm.

2. "Teenage Junk Food Is Bad for Your Junk," Menfertility.org, September 4, 2019, https://menfertility.org/teenage-junk-food-is-bad-for-your-junk/.

3. Y. H. Chiu et al., "Fruit and Vegetable Intake and Their Pesticide Residues in Relation to Semen Quality among Men from a Fertility Clinic," *Human Reproduction* 30, no. 6 (June 2015): 1342–51, https://academic.oup.com/humrep/article/30/6/1342/616110.

4. Carrie Madormo, "How Does Sperm Morphology Affect Fertility?" HealthLine, August 2, 2017, https://www.healthline.com/health/sperm-morphology.

5. "So Your Sperm Morphology Is Low—Should You Be Worried?" Fertility Solutions, https://fertilitysolutions.com.au/so-your-sperm-morphology-is-low-should-you-be-worried/.

6. Chaunie Brusie, "What Is Sperm Motility and How Does It Affect Fertility?" HealthLine, May 22, 2017, https://www.healthline.com/health/fertility/sperm-motility.

7. Vickie Barnes, "Improving Sperm Motility to Increase Chances of Getting Pregnant," BabyHopes.com, April 27, 2019, https://www.babyhopes.com/blogs/fertility/improving-sperm-motility.

8. Mayo Clinic Staff, "Male Infertility," Mayo Clinic, September 20, 2018, https://www.mayoclinic.org/diseases-conditions/male-infertility/symptoms-causes/syc-20374773.

9. Dalene Barton, "Goji Antioxidants Shown Helpful for Male Infertility," Natural Fertility Info, January 7, 2019, https://natural-fertility-info.com/goji-antioxidants-shown-helpful-for-male-infertility.html.

10. Shona Murray, MD, "Should I Take Testosterone to Help My Fertility? . . . NO, NO, NO," Advanced Reproductive Medecine, University of Colorado, May 1, 2017, https://arm.coloradowomenshealth.com/doctors-blog/testosterone-infertility.

11. Atli Arnarson, "10 Ways to Boost Male Fertility and Increase Sperm Count," HealthLine, May 18, 2020, https://www.healthline.com/health/boost-male-fertility-sperm-count.

Chapter 7: Debating Male Infertility Claims

1. Office of Public Affairs, "No, Guys, Your Cellphone Is Not Making You Infertile," *Health Feed* (blog), University of Utah, June 19, 2014, https://healthcare.utah.edu/healthfeed/postings/2014/06/061914_cellphone-cause-infertility.php.

2. Chanel Dubofsky, "Do Cell Phones Really Impact Sperm Quality?" *A Modern Fertility Blog*, April 30, 2018, https://modernfertility.com/blog/sperm/.

3. University of Exeter, "Mobile Phones Negatively Affect Male Fertility, New Study Suggests," EurekAlert, June 9, 2014, https://www.eurekalert.org/pub_releases/2014-06/uoe-mpn060914.php.

4. Paul Chisholm, "Boxers or Briefs? Experts Disagree Over Tight Underwear's Effect on Male Fertility," NPR, August 8, 2018, https://www.npr.org/sections/health-shots/2018/08/08/636901101/boxers-or-briefs-experts-disagree-over-tight-underwears-effect-on-male-fertility.

Chapter 8: When Advice Doesn't Help

1. Chris Iliades, MD, "Why Boozing Can Be Bad for Your Sex Life," Everyday Health, January 4, 2012, https://www.everydayhealth.com/erectile-dysfunction/why-boozing-can-be-bad-for-your-sex-life.aspx.

2. "Robitussin for Fertility FAQ," Fairhaven Health, https://www.fairhavenhealth.com/cm/.

3. Nicola, "Fertility and IVF Myths, Debunked," Access Fertility, September 25, 2019, https://www.accessfertility.com/blog/ivf-myths-debunked/.

4. Jen Gunter, MD, "7 Fertility Myths That Belong in the Past," *New York Times*, April 15, 2020, https://www.nytimes.com/2020/04/15/parenting/fertility /trying-to-conceive-myths.html.

5. Lauren Vinopal, "Female Orgasms Don't Help with Fertility. Here's Why the Myth Persists," Fatherly, August 28, 2019, https://www.fatherly.com /health-science/female-orgasms-conception-fertility-science/.

6. Department of Health and Human Services, "Age and Fertility," Better Health Channel, Victorian Government, February 28, 2014, https://www .betterhealth.vic.gov.au/health/conditionsandtreatments/age-and -fertility.

Chapter 9: Everything's Little with Sperm Tests

1. Rachel Gurevich, RN, "Problems Ejaculating for Semen Analysis," Verywell Family, September 17, 2020, https://www.verywellfamily.com/problems -ejaculating-for-a-semen-sample-1960162.

Chapter 10: Sex and Drugs

1. Amy Marturana Winderl, "6 Ways Infertility Impacts a Relationship," *Self*, May 20, 2016, https://www.self.com/story/how-infertility-impacts-a-couples -relationship.

2. Serena Chen, MD, "Are Your Chances of Getting Pregnant Better if You Have Sex in the Morning?" BabyCenter, https://www.babycenter.com/getting -pregnant/how-to-get-pregnant/are-your-chances-of-getting-pregnant -better-if-you-have-sex_1334780.

3. "Femara (Letrozole) for Infertility, Ovulation Problems, and PCOS Treatment," Advanced Fertility Center of Chicago, http://www.advancedfertility .com/femara-letrozole-fertility.htm.

4. "Male Fertility Drugs," University of Utah Health Care, https://healthcare .utah.edu/fertility/treatments/male-fertility-drugs.php.

5. Ohad Shoshany, MD, et al., "Outcomes of Anastrozole in Oligozoospermic Hypoandrogenic Subfertile Men," *Fertility and Sterility* 107, no. 3 (March 1, 2017): 589–94, https://doi.org/10.1016/j.fertnstert.2016.11.021.

Chapter 11: The Comedy of Infertility

1. Lora Shahine, "Infertility Is No Joke, but Sometimes You Just Need to Laugh," blog post, March 31, 2018, http://lorashahine.com/blog/2018/3/31/infer tility-is-no-joke-but-sometimes-you-just-need-to-laugh.

Chapter 12: Standing Strong in Marriage

1. Erica Berman, "When Infertility Affects Your Marriage," *HuffPost*, January 23, 2014, https://www.huffingtonpost.ca/erica-berman/infertility-and-depression_b_4251953.html.
2. Shannon Firth, "Study: Infertile Couples 3 Times More Likely to Divorce," *U.S. News & World Report*, January 30, 2014, https://www.usnews.com/news/articles/2014/01/31/study-infertile-couples-3-times-more-likely-to-divorce.
3. The text of this paragraph is paraphrased from an e-mail Kate Brian sent to me on March 24, 2020.

Chapter 13: Problem Solvers

1. Simon Niblock, "Men & the Problem with Being Problem Solvers," blog post, April 19, 2018, https://simonniblock.com/mens-roles/men-the-problem-with-being-problem-solvers/.
2. Rick Wamre, "Men Are Problem Solvers," *Oak Cliff Advocate*, August 1, 2006, https://oakcliff.advocatemag.com/2006/08/men-are-problem-solvers/.
3. Michelle Roya Rad, "10 Characteristics of Good Problem Solvers," *HuffPost*, November 24, 2014, https://www.huffpost.com/entry/problem-solving_b_4302935.
4. Celia Hoi Yan Chan et al., "Preferred Problem Solving and Decision-Making Role in Fertility Treatment among Women Following an Unsuccessful In Vitro Fertilization Cycle," *BMC Women's Health* 19, no. 153 (2019), https://doi.org/10.1186/s12905-019-0856-5.

Chapter 14: Men, Mental Health, and Infertility

1. Mayo Clinic Staff, "Male Depression: Understanding the Issues," Mayo Clinic, May 21, 2019, https://www.mayoclinic.org/diseases-conditions/depression/in-depth/male-depression/art-20046216.
2. Addiction.com Staff, "Five Substances That Can Affect Fertility," Addiction.com, February 22, 2015, https://www.addiction.com/blogs/substances-affect-fertility/.
3. James Elist, MD, "Infertile Men and Mental Health Issues," blog post, February 4, 2016, https://www.drelist.com/blog/infertile-men-mental-health-issues/.
4. Phil Christman, "What Is It Like to Be a Man?" *Hedgehog Review*, summer 2018, https://hedgehogreview.com/issues/identitieswhat-are-they-good-for/articles/what-is-it-like-to-be-a-man.

5. John Haltiwanger, "What It Means to 'Be a Man' in Today's World," *Elite Daily*, March 6, 2015, https://www.elitedaily.com/life/culture/what-means-to-be-a-man/958158.

Chapter 15: Avoid Being a Fertility Fool

1. Meghan Collie, "'Fertility Isn't Funny': Why You Shouldn't Pretend to Be Pregnant on April Fools' Day," Global News, April 1, 2019, https://globalnews.ca/news/5117058/pregnancy-prank-april-fools-day-joke-fertility-infertility/.
2. RMACT Team, "April Fool's Day—Funny Doesn't Have to Hurt," Reproductive Medicine Associates of Connecticut, March 29, 2018, https://www.rmact.com/fertility-blog/april-fools-day-funny-doesnt-have-to-hurt.

Chapter 16: The Religious View

1. "Fertility Issues: Sikh Arguments for and against Fertility Treatments," Bitesize, BBC, https://www.bbc.co.uk/bitesize/guides/z9kjpv4/revision/4.
2. Jane R. W. Fisher and Karin Hammarberg, "Psychological and Social Aspects of Infertility in Men: An Overview of the Evidence and Implications for Psychologically Informed Clinical Care and Future Research," *Asian Journal of Andrology* 14, no. 1 (January 2012): 121–29, https://www.ncbi.nlm.nih.gov/pmc/articles/PMC3735147/.
3. Mohammed Ali Al-Bar and Hassan Chamsi-Pasha, "Assisted Reproductive Technology: Islamic Perspective," in *Contemporary Bioethics* (Cham, Switzerland: Springer Nature, 2015), 173–86, https://doi.org/10.1007/978-3-319-18428-9_11.
4. Roy Homburg et al., "Religious Attitudes to Fertility: A Hindu View," Fertility Plus, July 12, 2018, https://www.fertilityplus.org.uk/religious-attitudes-to-fertility-a-hindu-view/.
5. "Guide to Buddhism A to Z," BuddhismA2Z.com, http://buddhisma2z.com/.

Chapter 17: Remember the Grandparents

1. Anna van Praagh, "The Generation Who May Never Be Grandparents," *Telegraph*, January 16, 2016, https://www.telegraph.co.uk/family/grandparents/the-generation-who-may-never-be-grandparents/.
2. Sharon N. Covington and Linda Hammer Burns, PhD, "When Infertility Strikes the Family: Helping the System Cope," Shady Grove Fertility, https://www.shadygrovefertility.com/emotional-support-articles/when-infertility-strikes.

Chapter 18: Not-so-Happy Father's Day

1. Remy Melina, "Father's Day Turns 100: How Did It Begin?" Live Science, June 17, 2010, https://www.livescience.com/10697-father-day-turns-100.html.
2. Spencer Blake, "What Father's Day Is Like when You're Struggling with Infertility," *Time*, June 16, 2016, https://time.com/4368232/fathers-day-infertility/.

Chapter 19: Our Furry Children

1. Greg Sdeo, "Goodbye Lila Hello Rupert," *A Few Pieces Missing from Normalcy—An Infertile Man's Perspective* (blog), July 20, 2019, https://afewpiecemissingfromnormalcy.wordpress.com/.

Chapter 20: Adoption and Other Options

1. Karla King, "Why Is the Adoption Rate Dropping?" Adoption.org, https://adoption.org/adoption-rate-dropping.
2. "Moving from Infertility to Adoption," Canada Adopts!, http://www.canadaadopts.com/hoping-adopt/moving-infertility-adoption/.
3. "Prohibitions Related to Surrogacy," Health Canada, February 5, 2020, https://www.canada.ca/en/health-canada/services/drugs-health-products/biologics-radiopharmaceuticals-genetic-therapies/legislation-guidelines/assisted-human-reproduction/prohibitions-related-surrogacy.html.
4. William Houghton, "Surrogacy in the United States," Sensible Surrogacy Guide, https://www.sensiblesurrogacy.com/surrogacy-in-the-united-states/.
5. "Frequently Asked Questions," Miracle Surrogacy, https://miraclesurrogacy.com/frequently-asked-questions/.

Chapter 21: Coping with Childlessness

1. Bibi Lynch, "Male Childlessness: 'You Think, If I'm Not Reproducing—Then What Am I?'" *Guardian*, November 17, 2018, https://www.theguardian.com/lifeandstyle/2018/nov/17/male-childlessness-not-reproducing-what-am-i.
2. Mila van Huis and Elma Wobma, "More Childless Men," Statistics Netherlands (CBS), July 6, 2010, https://www.cbs.nl/en-gb/news/2010/27/more-childless-men.

Chapter 25: Seeking Kinship (aka Dude, Where's My Infertile Tribe?)

1. Samantha Philips, "15 Reasons Why Men Don't Talk about Their Feelings . . . ," AllWomensTalk.com, July 18, 2020, https://allwomenstalk.com/top-secrets-why-men-dont-talk-about-their-feelings/.

2. Cindi May, "Are Women More Emotionally Expressive Than Men?" *Scientific American*, August 30, 2017, https://www.scientificamerican.com/article /are-women-more-emotionally-expressive-than-men/.

3. Nikelle Murphy, "Science Explains Why Women Talk More Than Men," Showbiz Cheat Sheet, September 20, 2015, https://www.cheatsheet.com /health-fitness/science-explains-why-women-talk-more-than-men.html/.

Chapter 26: I-U-AYE

1. "Intrauterine Insemination: IUI," American Pregnancy Association, April 24, 2017, https://americanpregnancy.org/getting-pregnant/intrauterine -insemination/.

2. Rachel Gurevich, RN, "Is IUI a Successful Fertility Treatment?" Verywell Family, October 2, 2020, https://www.verywellfamily.com/what-is-the-iui -success-rate-1960191.

3. Aimee Eyvazzadeh, MD, "Why Isn't Your IUI Working?" *Medium*, November 22, 2019, https://medium.com/@eggwhisperer/why-isnt-your-iui -working-5c9123332050.

Chapter 27: The Complete Idiot's Guide to IVF

1. "IVF by the Numbers," *Fertility Blog*, Penn Medicine, March 14, 2018, https:// www.pennmedicine.org/updates/blogs/fertility-blog/2018/march/ivf-by -the-numbers.

2. "What Is Intracytoplasmic Sperm Injection (ICSI)?" ReproductiveFacts.org, 2014, https://www.reproductivefacts.org/news-and-publications/patient -fact-sheets-and-booklets/documents/fact-sheets-and-info-booklets /what-is-intracytoplasmic-sperm-injection-icsi/.

Chapter 28: The Road You Travel for Fertility

1. Megan Leonhardt, "Women Are Traveling Far and Wide for Affordable IVF— Here's Why It's so Expensive," CNBC, August 13, 2019, https://www.cnbc .com/2019/08/13/women-are-traveling-far-and-wide-for-affordable-ivf .html.

2. CTVNews.ca Staff, "Some Canadians Turning to Sun-Soaked Foreign Fertility Clinics for 'Procreation Vacations,'" CTV News, April 8, 2018, https:// www.ctvnews.ca/health/some-canadians-turning-to-sun-soaked-foreign -fertility-clinics-for-procreation-vacations-1.3876091.

Chapter 29: The Second Miscarriage and Secondary Infertility

1. Margaret Renkl, "'We Can't Get Pregnant Again,'" *Parents*, October 5, 2005, https://www.parents.com/pregnancy/considering-baby/another/we-cant-get-pregnant-again/.

2. Charles Coddington, MD, "Secondary Infertility: Why Does It Happen?" Mayo Clinic, January 30, 2020, https://www.mayoclinic.org/diseases-conditions/infertility/expert-answers/secondary-infertility/faq-20058272.

3. Generations Fertility Care, "Secondary Infertility," University of Wisconsin Hospitals and Clinics Authority, https://www.uwhealth.org/infertility/secondary-infertility/25058.

4. Sharon Mazel, "Secondary Infertility," What to Expect, September 10, 2020, https://www.whattoexpect.com/getting-pregnant/fertility/secondary-infertility/.

Chapter 30: It Doesn't Go Away

1. Windy Ezzell, "The Impact of Infertility on Women's Mental Health," *North Carolina Medical Journal* 77, no. 6 (November 2016): 427–28, https://doi.org/10.18043/ncm.77.6.427.

About the Author

Jon **Waldman** is a writer and author based in Winnipeg, Manitoba, Canada, where he lives with his wife, Elana; their daughter, Kaia; and their dog, Mercer. Jon earned his BA at the University of Winnipeg and his MJ through Ryerson University's post-graduate journalism program, and began his career as a freelancer with publications such as the *Winnipeg Free Press*, the *Winnipeg Sun*, the *Toronto Sun*, *Winnipeg Men* magazine, the *Hockey News*, and others. He has since been featured in several print and online publications, including blogs, as part of his career in marketing and communications.

Jon's first venture into the book world came in 2009 when he coedited *Slam! Wrestling: Shocking Stories from the Squared Circle*. From there, Jon cowrote *Got 'Em, Got 'Em, Need 'Em: A Fan's Guide to Collecting the Top 100 Sports Cards of All Time* (2011) before publishing his first solo effort, *He Shoots, He Saves: The Story of Hockey's Collectible Treasures*, in 2015. Later that year, he published *100 Things Jets Fans Should Know & Do Before They Die*, which was a top seller in Winnipeg for several months and was short-listed for the Carol Shields Winnipeg Book Award in 2016.

Jon began his path as an infertility advocate in 2014, giving his first interview with CJOB in Winnipeg. Since then, he has been interviewed by CBC, CTV, Global TV, *HuffPost*, and others. In 2017, Jon delivered his first TEDx Talk, called "Swimming Aimlessly: Getting Men to Talk about Infertility," and has also spoken during the UK's National Infertility Awareness Week. Jon is a past board member of Fertility Matters Canada and now serves on their advisory committee. He and Elana have also spoken privately with several individuals and couples who have been on their own infertility journeys.

Outside of work, Jon enjoys spending time with his family, biking, and watching documentaries. Contact him on Twitter @JonWaldman or on Instagram @Jon_Waldman.